More praise for

Happy Healthy Gut

"*Happy Healthy Gut* is a necessary read for all. Jennifer Browne not only provides effective solutions for those suffering from digestive disorders, but provides the link between gut health and optimal health, encouraging everyone to feel their absolute best! Browne filters through all the crap (pun intended) and provides insight and education in a way that's approachable, direct and fun to read!"

—Peggy Kotsopoulos, Registered Holistic Nutritionist
and author of *Must Have Been Something I Ate*

"*Happy Healthy Gut* is an immensely important read for people who love food, but struggle with IBS and other gastrointestinal sensitivities. Browne offers a well thought out argument for adopting a plant-based diet as a step towards improved quality of life. This book engenders a sense of control in those trying to negotiate medical systems not well set up for managing complex symptoms where medication and surgical interventions fall short."

—Dr. Jesse Sidhu BSc MD FRCP(C) MPH Acute and Consultant Liaison
Psychiatrist Clinical Instructor Department of Psychiatry;
UBC, Vancouver

"Inspiring and informative; Jennifer takes you through her digestive journey, while educating her readers about the digestive system and the impact a plant-based diet can have on it. I love finding a book such as this one, that brings a true recovery story into the spotlight. The masses need to know that we can become responsible for our health, natural remedies do work, and reversing dis-ease is possible! Thanks for sharing your experiences with us, Jen!"

—Stephanie Ablett, CNP
Certified Holistic Nutritionist and Vegan Food Enthusiast
www.naturalginger.ca

Happy Healthy Gut

The Plant-Based Diet Solution to Curing IBS and Other Chronic Digestive Disorders

Jennifer Browne

SKYHORSE PUBLISHING

Skyhorse Publishing books may be purchased in bulk at special discounts for sales promotion, corporate gifts, fund-raising, or educational purposes. Special editions can also be created to specifications. For details, contact the Special Sales Department, Skyhorse Publishing, 307 West 36th Street, 11th Floor, New York, NY 10018 or info@skyhorsepublishing.com.

Skyhorse® and Skyhorse Publishing® are registered trademarks of Skyhorse Publishing, Inc.®, a Delaware corporation.

Visit our website at www.skyhorsepublishing.com.

10 9 8 7 6 5 4 3 2 1

Library of Congress Cataloging-in-Publication Data

Browne, Jennifer (Jennifer Shay), 1981-
 Happy healthy gut : the natural diet solution to curing IBS and other chronic digestive disorders / Jennifer Browne.
    pages cm
 Includes bibliographical references and index.
 ISBN 978-1-62636-041-9 (alk. paper)
 1. Irritable colon--Diet therapy--Recipes. 2. Irritable colon--Treatment--Popular works. 3. Colon (Anatomy)--Diseases--Nutritional aspects--Popular works. I. Title.
 RC862.I77B76 2014
 616.3'42--dc23
                    2013032405

Paperback ISBN: 978-1-63450-673-1
E-book ISBN: 978-1-62873-831-5

Cover design by Jane Sheppard
Author photo by Cristal Sawatzky, Level 6 Images
Cover photo: iStock/Thinkstock
Printed in the United States of America

Acknowledgments

Thanks to my supportive friends and family, who, after being informed I was taking this project on, didn't laugh or scoff at me. Not even once.

Many thanks to Judy, Kim, Kelly, Jeff, and Marie for sharing their personal experiences with digestive disaster and triumph. Your stories are empowering, and I hope they will help others.

My sincere gratitude to Ann, whose meticulous edits on this book could not be more appreciated. Thank you.

Lastly, to Seventh Avenue Literary and Skyhorse Publishing: thank you for believing in this book.

Dedication

To the massive population of people who suffer from digestive disorders: don't give up, and don't settle for anything less than your ideal situation. Strive for fabulous health, and you'll get there. Be your own best advocate.

For my husband Dave, who has seemingly unlimited patience with me; my mom and Ashlee, who are always quietly inspirational; my dad, whose motivation and drive did not go unnoticed, and my children, who did not seem to mind being ignored while this book was being written. (Seriously—you three are *really* good at entertaining yourselves.)

I love you all.

CONTENTS

Preface

"The food you eat can either be the safest and most powerful form of medicine, or the slowest form of poison."[1]

—Dr. Ann Wigmore, pioneer for natural health

How many times have your feet been sore, yet you continue to stand? What about feeling exhausted all the time? Do you make more time for quality sleep, or just make another pot of coffee? That new mother who is still tender from delivery—is she taking the time to rest, or is she doing housework and entertaining within hours of welcoming her new baby? When you have consistent heartburn when you eat pizza, do you stop eating it, or do you simply treat your symptoms with a handful of antacids?

What about cheese, a processed bun, or a steak? Does your stomach scream at you after eating these things? If so, do you listen?

The floor is not your friend, and you shouldn't have to cling to it every time your bowel feels like escaping the rest of your body. It's amazing how you can live for decades before becoming aware that the direction in which your life is headed is just not good enough for you. You simply decide one day that you want your life to change, *need* it to change, and you suddenly feel that you must begin this transformation immediately.

And so you do.

I want to be clear about my objective for writing this book. After nearly ten years of moderate stomach pain due to irritable bowel syndrome (IBS), which I was diagnosed with in my early twenties, I finally discovered what makes it stop, and it took little time and almost no effort. It also worked for a handful of other digestive disorder sufferers that I was in communication with throughout the duration of writing this book. I'm not talking about drugs, radical treatments, or experimental surgeries. I'm talking about diet: specifically, a whole food, plant-based diet. By fully integrating this type of dietary platform into my daily regimen, I have improved my quality of life in ways I never even thought possible, and so have others. Together we have transformed from robots, who put up with daily digestive discomfort, to men and women who have refused a mediocre life and so began a new one, full of endless possibilities in the Land of Great Digestive Ease.

Who knew such a place existed?!

If you are living with a digestive disorder, then you already know that symptoms change, and that the individual situations that can set off bowel reactions can be unexpectedly altered, too. I know many people living with IBS, and although I'm sure what we experience is similar, it is never exactly the same, and even the triggers can change from person to person, day to day. The simple idea of food having the ability to cure all of these variations in digestive discomfort can spark considerable skepticism. However, when you consider all that entails in introducing a whole, varied, earthy, plant-based plan into your life, it only makes perfect sense that it should work.

And it does.

A key component to attaining digestive success with this plan is to acknowledge the slight, yet important distinction between the terms "vegetarian" and "plant-based." Although both descriptions imply the ridding of animal products from your diet, one can certainly be an unhealthy vegetarian. Just because you don't eat ground beef, doesn't mean you don't eat high-fat, low-nutrient food. You can't just simply eliminate animal products to jump on this bandwagon headed to Digestive Bliss Town; you must forgo the insanely ridiculous amount of fake products that surround us, and introduce many new foods into your life. Expand your vegetable base, discover new grains, and learn techniques for fermenting, sprouting, and juicing your food.

Adopting a new and amazing way to think about food shows that you have an active opinion about your health, and that you refuse to let digestive discomfort rule your life. It's also about purging your poor body of all those bad foods you've been feeding it for years. I'm not blaming you! We live in an age of incredible convenience, variety, and availability, while also being deprived of basic knowledge regarding the subject of what our food is really composed of.

You can go to your local grocer and buy a pineapple in January. Do you know where that pineapple is from or how it got here? That chicken you might be having for dinner has come from an average of 1500 miles away, and is full of all things genetically modified, which can hardly be recognized as food. The process of getting that poultry to your plate is a procedure few of us are aware of, and, because of that, we have no idea how it might be hurting us.

This book is about teaching you, the Intestinally Distressed, how to make amazing nutritional choices that will help your whole self glow while your tummy celebrates, shouting "free at last!" We only get one body, and we must live with it for close to a century. By learning how to treat it like the temple it is, it will thank you in numerous and glorious ways, including giving you the gift of cessation of digestive pain.

What I want to do throughout the course of this book, is simply share all that I have learned as it pertains to diet and detriment, and hope that it appeals to others who have experienced, or are currently experiencing, chronic pain and/or disease, as well as those who are simply looking to make a positive change in their diet and spirit. I want to introduce to you the facts about our "western diet" so that you can make your own choice as to whether or not you need to make a lifestyle change.

Whole food, plant-based eating is not about making it difficult to grocery shop, and the goal is definitely not to stir up frustration, so that you run straight to the closest burger joint. It's a journey that opens your mind, changes your opinions, coyly introduces you to your own body, demands that you more closely examine how you want to live your life, and educates you how to accomplish doing this pain free. This lifestyle decision began as a quest to stop my stomach pain, but it has turned out to be an incredible force that continues to heal me in countless ways, with the absence of chronic pain being a small part of the entire mosaic. I am by no means an expert in any medical field, but I do know firsthand what this platform for better health has the power to do, and for that I am so grateful.

As a fabulous by-product of adopting a whole food, plant-based diet, you'll learn how changing your eating habits will help you not only greatly improve your own quality of life, but also effortlessly contribute to many other causes, such as saving some animals, helping direct food back to the hungry, and improving the current condition of our suffering planet. The blatant disregard for human health that has become synonymous with farmed animal welfare is astonishing, and it is my desire to pass along important knowledge to you about food issues that are rarely discussed and/or thought about, and why these matters have plenty to do with today's enormous influx of digestive despair.

While there is plenty of information available to the public regarding the anatomy of the human digestive tract and its tendency to be unpredictable and confusing, there isn't enough attainable research that questions why certain components of our food might be the leading cause of digestive disorders. Issues such as genetic modification, food irradiation, chemical additives, and mass-scale factory-farmed livestock products are a few of the topics that are discussed in this book. Doesn't it make sense to consider altered food as a major player in the game of digestive roulette? I decided to step outside of the box in my own quest to discover what contributed to my own digestive malfunction, and was surprised by the results. Though research may be close to nil regarding the safety and long-term effects that such foodstuffs may have on our bodies, this doesn't mean that we can't investigate for ourselves, and start discovering now if something seemingly innocent is messing with our digestive tracts.

We need to take it upon ourselves to start thinking "food-forward"—to critically recognize whether or not any given food will contribute to our overall growth and escalating health, or if it will simply satisfy our immediate caloric needs, and promote disease and digestive malfunction.

This book is the compilation all of the knowledge I have accumulated, and encompasses absolutely everything I have found personally constructive and useful in my journey to good digestive health. It is about aiding you to find out why the food you are choosing to consume may be the root cause of the digestive discomfort and other health issues that you may be enduring and how, by taking the proverbial bull by its horns, you can take huge steps towards improving your own digestive health without the need for medications and surgeries, while simultaneously bypassing general affliction and impairment. A whole food, plant-based plan can change your entire life. If you feel that your time for a tune-up has come, whether for better health, a clearer mind, or in order to take responsibility for today's heady ethical or environmental issues, then you've come to the right place.

I hope your journey is enlightening, positive and, with little effort, pain free. Let me show you how to get your life back quickly, because you've already spent too much time feeling like crap.

Let your journey to great digestive health begin . . .

Part 1

The Why (The Problem)

The first section of this book is all about problems. The issues we're facing as a nation with inadequate digestion, the obstacles our digestive systems have with attempting to process foods that our bodies can't handle, and the dilemmas that arise when we try and force ourselves to ignore an ongoing issue that can (and will) only get worse.

It will provide an accurate description of the digestive process, introduce you to a handful of common digestive diseases, and discuss inflammation, the health concerns associated with consuming animal products, reductionism, food-borne disease, genetic modification, food irradiation, and more. It was written with education in mind, and with the intention of convincing you why adopting a whole food, plant-based platform provides a clear path to good digestive health. By knowing what you're up against in terms of the quality of food that is being made available to you, you can then proceed to implement better decision making in regards to your grocery list. The following is the low-down on what is happening with our food to which we might not be paying attention, and items that you may be consuming on a daily basis that are probable contributors to your digestive unease.

Chapter 1

To Tame a Tummy . . .

"Nothing's changed my life more. I feel better about myself as a person, being conscious and responsible for my actions and I lost weight and my skin cleared up and I got bright eyes and I just became stronger and healthier and happier. Can't think of anything better in the world to be but be vegan."[2]
—Alicia Silverstone, actress, activist, and vegan foodie

As it was, I became used to missing birthdays, parties, weddings, and work. I was so deep into feeling unwell that I completely forgot what it was like to feel normal. You just get used to feeling terrible, and then once you experience the normalcy of a perfectly working digestive system again, after nine years, it's akin to the feeling of waking up one day forty pounds lighter, after attempting to lose it for nearly a decade. For me, it was as simple as a clicking sound that resonated throughout my brain one random day, like any other, at my mother's house.

Luckily for me (and not so much my husband), I'm like a crow: I like shiny things. It's weird how sometimes all it takes is something very small and unassuming to get your internal pendulum swinging in a different direction. One of the most important life decisions I have ever made for myself began by catching a glimpse of a sparkly bracelet (the shiny thing) lying on top of a book I saw on my mom's kitchen counter in October of 2010. After trying to convince myself that I owned many bracelets, that I didn't need this particular one, and that I should probably check into some sort of shopping rehab, my attention turned to the book. It immediately had me curious because it had Alicia Silverstone's name listed as the author, and I didn't know she was a writer. I flipped through it for five minutes, and even though it was clear that my mom was only half way through reading it, I "asked" her to lend it to me, and I whisked it home.

Silverstone's *The Kind Diet* was the first of several books on plant-based eating that I ended up reading that month, and by November, I had completely changed my mind about food and food animals. These books marked the beginning of my love affair with healthy food, and the end of my decade-long problem with (and I'm putting this nicely) inadequate digestion.

Here's how it all went down:

Growing up, I always considered my family to be pretty healthy eaters. My mom (who's totally embarrassed by this) does admit to orchestrating tea parties with my sister and I that consisted of artificially flavored drinks and candy, but she also went through the trouble of making all of our meals, and we never ate out. During those tea party days, I even remember being force-fed tablespoons of cod liver oil. You know, along with the candy. We had a balanced diet . . .

When I was twenty, I was diagnosed (after several invasive exploratory procedures including laparoscopies, colonoscopies, and one very unpleasant and predictably shocking barium enema), with irritable bowel syndrome, otherwise known as IBS.

My symptoms were bloating, gas, chronic constipation, stomach pain, and chronic back pain. By-products of these symptoms were hemorrhoids, insomnia, weight gain, and occasional depression. Sounds super fun, right? Sometimes my symptoms were so bad that

I would only be able to walk hunched over, and occasionally the episodes would last for days or even weeks.

IBS is a diagnosis of exclusion, which doctors like to give to people when they can't figure out why their digestive tracts aren't working properly. Approximately seventy million Americans suffer from digestive disorders like IBS,[3] with almost twenty percent of the U.S. population exhibiting IBS-like symptoms.[4] Canada's number? 20 million.[5] That's pretty prevalent! Basically, we are told that there is always medication and steroids to help with the pain and symptoms if they get out of control. I'm very certain that this sounds familiar to many of you. When you consider that there are currently about 315 million people living in the United States,[6] then that means that one out of four and a half people suffer from a debilitating disease that I now know is completely repairable and reversible.

I thought nothing of my diagnosis at the time. I was young and relieved that the exploratory procedure portion of my early twenties was finally over. It didn't occur to me to persistently ask any of the doctors I had seen any questions about IBS, or what it meant for my future, and they didn't offer up very much information. The name sounded innocent enough: irritable bowel syndrome. Like my stomach was cranky, but similar to anyone who is going through a particularly moody or self-proclaimed depressed period in their life, my abdomen would eventually get over it and carry on as if nothing happened. You know, like immature teenage angst.

Well, that didn't happen, and so I waded through the next nine and a half years trying to hide my pain and bloating, while desperately searched for anything that made me feel more human and less zombie. It was very scary. At one point, I actually remember telling my mom that I was convinced I would end up with colon cancer. Although I never considered trying any of the available medication prescribed for IBS (because I've always been a holistic kind of girl), I did find some things helpful like peppermint and fennel essential oils. I used to rub them all over my stomach when I could feel an episode coming, and sometimes that would help to mellow my symptoms. Hot towels placed directly over my lower abdomen would work sometimes, too. I also discovered that if I laid flat on my back on a hard floor it would assist in decreasing the bloating and pain, as long as I wasn't too far gone. (And as long I was at home, of course!) Things like sitting for hours (particularly flying) would guarantee to commence stomach pain. My husband knew that when we landed at our destination, I would have to walk hunched over to our hotel room with my pants unbuttoned because of the incredible bloating, and then would have to lie down as soon as possible. Just for the record, this was not just any old bloating. I totally looked like I was five months pregnant when this would happen. It was embarrassing and very stressful, which made my symptoms even worse. I remember teaching English as a Second Language (ESL) for a particularly precocious group of children one year, and a couple of the girls constantly asking me if I was expecting a baby. (Seven and eight-year-olds have no boundaries, and certainly no tact.) Needless to say, I was extremely self-conscious.

Did I mention that I was a complete laxative addict? I knew that it wasn't healthy to take laxatives all the time, and that it would be bad for me to become addicted to them, so in my warped way of thinking, I thought it would be better to incorporate different brands and types into my routine. I rotated between Senna tablets, Metamucil, and Dieter's Green Tea in the hopes that I wouldn't become dependent on one or all of them permanently. (The logic was not sound.) I did the laxative dance for about eight years, and it was common for me to not move my bowels for five to seven days at a stretch, which I now know was so incredibly bad for me.

In my early twenties, my diet consisted of lots of creamy white pastas, bagels with cream cheese, cheese sandwiches, and crackers and cheese. (As you've probably already noted, I love cheese. It's my crack.) I was in university, and those were my comfort foods. I also drank a lot of wine, and ate huge portions at every mealtime. Even though I thought I was pretty healthy, my diet was a disaster waiting to happen. I would habitually work out five days a week (for years), and not drop a pound.

Around the age of twenty-three (still relatively early in my IBS days), I accidentally stumbled upon the fact that, much to my severe disappointment, wheat products made me feel generally inflamed. When I abstained from them, I did not have as many IBS symptoms. In fact, for my wedding at the age of twenty-four, I didn't eat any breads or pasta for three months before the big day for fear that I would get bloated in my very tight wedding dress. I pretty much gave up bagels, pasta, and pizza, in their entirety, until I was twenty-nine. On the odd time when I did eat those things, I paid for it dearly and swiftly. The initial discovery about the wheat products was my first inclination that food going in played a pretty big role in how I felt, as did what came out. When I stopped eating wheat for my wedding, I effortlessly dropped close to ten pounds within a span of three or four months. No wonder Dr. Atkins had so many followers! The thing is, as soon as I went back to eating wheat, my stomach resumed its daily rant, and I gained back the weight. If I tried to go completely carb-free, I got completely exhausted and very moody. It sucked, and I was getting depressed.

My paternal grandfather died of complications due to celiac disease (an autoimmune disease characterized by the inability to tolerate gluten), so I started to think that maybe I had inherited that; but celiac disease was ruled out through a blood test and a small biopsy of my colon. Twice. I was also paying more attention to the fact that my symptoms were not just wheat-related. In fact, for lack of a more refined description, I noticed that they completely correlated with the frequency of my bowel movements! If I was regular, like when I abstained from wheat, I felt good and lost weight. If I was constipated, like I was most of the time, I felt terrible and I gained weight. In other words, I realized that in order to ward off symptoms, I needed to remain consistent in the bathroom. Ditching the wheat helped, but not enough for me to stop investigating and call it a day. By now, I had three children, and I was sick and tired of being sick and tired. I needed energy, stamina, and a real fix for my stupid IBS, and I needed it right away.

When I started reading about what a plant-based diet had to offer, and it was explained to me that meat is very heavy, tough to digest, acidic, inflammatory and disease provoking, a light went on in my head. I'm so happy for the existence of that light! About a week after cutting out beef, pork, and poultry, I felt like a different person. I felt light, energised, and . . . regular! The laxatives were no longer part of my life after only one week, and the essential oils and random floor flops were gone too. And it didn't stop there. The longer I abstained from meat, the better I felt. In fact, I was able to reintroduce wheat-based foods to my meals with very few consequences. There was definitely something amazing about my new plant-strong diet.

Premature Evaluation: Some initial observances were predictable, but there were many that were rather surprising! For the first four or five days, I felt terrible. I thought that perhaps I had made a huge mistake. I had low energy, my skin started to break out, and my stomach actually felt more bloated than before. But overnight, around day six or seven, something shifted in my body and my stomach stopped hurting and bloating. I felt lighter, I had *way* more energy, I became totally regular, and I felt calmer than ever. In the next few months, I also noticed that my skin got better and brighter, I lost weight, and my menstrual cycle regulated, the result being lighter and shorter periods. That last one was a huge bonus that I did not expect. Talk about motivation!

It's unfathomable how many millions of people put up with digestive trouble. Your digestive system is something that you use every single day, something that has the power to eradicate harmful bacteria, and absorb helpful nutrients. This system is complex and amazing, and given the right foods, it can be your closest ally. However, when you mistreat it by eating a typical western diet full of preserved, diseased, and overly processed ingredients, that same system has the ability to turn your entire world upside-down.

The craziest thing about our bodies is the ability we have to adapt. We are constantly changing within our environment, and our bodies do their best to adapt comfortably for us. When we push too much for too long, however, we are given signs to slow down or stop, though in our crazy, busy western world, we rarely listen. We are just not as in tune with ourselves as we should be, and we're paying for it by not taking a minute every now and then to listen to our bodies respond to us, whether to protest or to approve our actions.

We need to start honoring our bodies, listening to its protests, and adjusting our actions accordingly. I know it's hard. It took me a very long time to get to the point where I decided to listen (especially where cheese is concerned), but I'm so thankful I got here. I want you to get here, too. When you do, maybe you could congratulate yourself by springing for something shiny . . .

Question: Do you really listen to your body, or do you tune it out because you're just tired of hearing it complain? By finding a new entry point to solving your digestive issue, such as adopting a healthy platform for building better digestion, perhaps you can get it to stop screaming, and just calmly tell you what's wrong. Then, take the opportunity to fix the actual problem, not just deal with isolated symptoms.

Chapter 2

Digestion 101

Although most people don't consciously think about digestion on a regular basis (unless you have a digestive disorder, and therefore are aware of it constantly), this process affects our entire body every minute of every day. If anything interrupts this very intricate process, it can become disastrous for us on an immediate level (like food poisoning), or on a slower, more gradual, but potentially more serious level (like chronic disease). When I first began researching the digestive process and what it entailed, I was very surprised by my lack of even rudimentary knowledge on the subject. This incredibly important, key aspect to everyday living was so much more complex than I had originally thought. So, in an effort to pass on some basic digestion education, this chapter is dedicated to helping you understand your digestive system, and why the food we eat can affect so much of our internal, delicate balance.

Most people assume (like I did) that digestion begins in the stomach, but it actually commences the second food or drink enters your mouth, or even before that, if you get a good enough whiff of something tasty. The saliva that is produced when you smell good food or begin to eat is designed to produce two essential enzymes, used for breaking down carbohydrates (amylase), and fat (lipase).

These enzymes need to be thoroughly mixed with food in order to be effective, so that means you have to chew your food really well. Just by chewing better, you can help your body digest more easily.

When you swallow, the food travels down your esophagus. The esophageal sphincter is like a trap door that opens to allow food into your stomach, and then closes to prevent food from going back up. Those who have trouble with GERD (chronic acid reflux) often have problems with this muscle opening too easily and allowing food back up into the throat. Babies may also have a little trouble with this in the first few months, which is why it seems that they love to spit their food up.

Once your food has reached your stomach (which is probably higher up than you think), it is combined with hydrochloric acid and pepsinogen, which help to break down the proteins in your food into amino acids, and also help with the absorption of certain minerals. While all this is happening, your stomach is producing mucous (yeah, I said mucous) to help coat its lining, which prevents it from being eaten raw by the highly concentrated hydrochloric acid, which can lead to ulcers. This acid is extremely important to the digestive process, because while it's helping to break down proteins, it's also killing harmful bacteria that may have entered your body via the food that you just swallowed. An example of one such bacterium that everyone has heard of is *E. coli*.

Too little acid can result in an overgrowth of dangerous bacteria, which can flourish in the gut. Small children and elderly people are often at greater risk of more serious complications due to food-borne disease, because they don't produce as much of this substance as older children and adults do.

Once the food in your stomach has been properly broken down and ready for transport, it's released from the stomach into the small intestine through another trap door. A series of contractions and relaxations is what pushes the food throughout the length of your small intestine, which is approximately twenty-three feet long. While your food is making its way through your small intestine, nutrients are being absorbed.

There are three main parts to the small intestine, each with its own important function. They are called the duodenum, jejunum and ileum.[7] (Whoever came up with these names clearly thought it would be funny to hear people say them.) The villi in the duodenum produce different enzymes to help break down sugar. Bile, which is made in the liver but stored in the gallbladder, is added to the liquefied food and helps to break down fats. Other enzymes created in the pancreas help break down carbohydrates, proteins, and fats even further. During the last ten feet of the small intestine (the ileum), proteins, carbohydrates, fats, vitamins, and minerals are absorbed as much as possible.

From the small intestine, a valve (another trap door!) opens up and allows the food to filter into the large intestine, or colon, and then closes. It also makes sure that the (now) fecal matter cannot flow backwards, back into the small intestine. IBS-like symptoms can occur if this valve malfunctions and allows the backwards flow of fecal matter, or if the mucosal layer has been damaged and permits the intestinal wall to become permeable. (This is commonly called "leaky gut syndrome.")[8]

Once our food is in the large intestine, water and more minerals are absorbed and the fecal matter gains bulk. There should be a large amount of "friendly" bacteria in the colon, which aids in the digestion of soluble fiber and produces various vitamins. The fecal matter hangs out in the rectum, and then we eliminate it through the . . . you know. Have I painted a pretty picture?

Ideally, your food should spend less than one day in your digestive tract. When the millions of bacteria that make up a portion of your stool are not removed through quick elimination, they create a lot of gas caused by the overabundance of growth in the short term, and can contribute to other health problems in the long term. Regular elimination is vital, and should not be under-estimated or under-appreciated.

In the western world, we seem to have this bad habit of sitting on the toilet for a long time during defecation. (Thank God I have children. Otherwise I would never be able to write words like this without turning bright red and emitting strange sounds of nervous laughter.) This situation creates a stressed bowel, and the emergence of new BFFs (best friends forever) called hemorrhoids.

These friends suck. It is *not* a reciprocal relationship.

Elimination should take us no longer than a couple of minutes, and ideally, less than one. You should not be straining. If you are, then you need to rethink your current diet, while you sip warm water with lemon and a pinch of cayenne pepper, in an effort to stimulate your bowels.

Our digestive system serves one major purpose—to absorb the nutrients in the food we eat, in order to keep us alive and not dying of malnutrition. Without food, there would be no need for digestion. The two (food and digestion) go hand-in-hand. So, wouldn't it be reasonable to assume that what we eat directly affects our digestive systems, and therefore us in our entirety?

Because there is a well-known brain-gut connection (it has been documented that we have approximately as many nerve endings in our stomachs as we do in our spinal cords), it is safe to conclude that stress plays an important role in digestion. In fact, the gut is thought to possess its own brain—this is called the enteric nervous system. It's theorized that during fetal development, the central nervous system (brain and spinal cord) and the enteric nervous system share the same clump of tissue, until that tissue divides and becomes two separate systems. It explains why anxiety, stress, and other emotions are so often felt in our stomachs.[9]

We also all know that there are many things that are bad for us to try and ingest, like poisonous plants, mouldy nuts and wormy apples. So, we leave those items alone and instead eat things that we presume our bodies can handle—things that we have been taught by our country's leading nutritionists to eat in order to stay healthy. But what if some of those things were actually really hurting us? We know that it can be lethal to eat a peanut if you have a peanut allergy, but what about food allergies or sensitivities that don't create such an extreme reaction? A fabulous example of this is lactose intolerance. There are millions of people out there who possess this intolerance and don't even know it. They think they have a digestive issue, such as IBS, or perhaps they think that they are just naturally extremely gassy. By eliminating dairy, they would eliminate their symptoms.

Another example is celiac disease, the inability to process gluten products properly. Products containing gluten (and there are alot of them) can cause major discomfort for people with this intolerance, but again, it is often misdiagnosed or completely overlooked. Gluten goes in, inflammation occurs, digestion is incomplete, and pain is the result. By eliminating wheat, and other gluten products, symptoms subside.

What about meat? When I take a bite of steak, a reaction occurs, and my digestive system stops cold. Nobody talks about a "meat allergy," or "meat intolerance," but that's exactly what I would describe this as. Animal products go in, my gut screams with a sudden inflammatory reaction, I bloat, I feel pain, and I skip a week's worth of bowel movements. So, in a reasonable response to this cycle, I finally just stopped eating meat. Voila! No pain.

Eliminating heavy meats can also work wonders for digestive disorder sufferers because many of us produce much less stomach acid than we should, particularly as we get older.[10] With not as much acid to help break down the hard-to-digest animal tissue, the meal just sits in your stomach for longer, waiting until it can be pushed on to the next stage of digestion. You know if you have low stomach acidity if your stool contains undigested food. If you are regularly noticing this, then take it as a sign to start aiding your digestive tract. It is obviously not doing the job it could or should be doing.

Question: Do you eliminate foods from your diet that you know bother your stomach? If not, why? Have you forgotten what it's like to consistently feel good, or are you taking a purposeful, defiant stance against this force that you feel you have no control over? You do have control. You also have willpower. You and your body are not separate entities. Help it, and you will be helped in return.

Chapter 3

The D.D. No One Wants Around

"In 2004, there were more than 236,000 deaths in the United States with a digestive disease as the underlying cause."[11]
—The Burden of Digestive Diseases in the United States

"To go or not to go?" is not the question. It's "can I go, or am I constipated?" Or, "I don't want to go, please make it stop!" Let's examine and define some of the more common digestive diseases that plague us here in the United States and Canada. I specify these two countries, because our ailments, although they sometimes overlap, are different from those in other areas of the world, particularly developing countries. In many developing countries, digestive problems are generally caused by such things as parasitic disease, tuberculosis, contaminated water, and malnutrition.[12] In North America, we suffer from what Dr. T. Colin Campbell, PhD and co-author of *The China Study*, calls "diseases of affluence,"[13] which are brought on usually by poor dietary choices, caused in most part by the high level of miscommunication and terrible nutrition education that we who live in North America are privy to.

Lucky us!

Although many of these diseases include diabetes, cancers, hypertension, obesity and coronary heart disease, I personally believe that digestive diseases could be added to this list of diseases of affluence as well. A somewhat comprehensive list of digestive diseases that are common in our region of the world include, in alphabetical order, "Barrett's esophagus, celiac disease, colon cancer, constipation, Crohn's disease, diarrhea, diverticular disease, dyspepsia, esophogeal cancer, GERD, gastric ulcers, inflammatory bowel disease, irritable bowel syndrome, lactose intolerance, pancreatitis, peptic ulcer, and ulcerative colitis."[14] (Whew!) I bet if you thought hard for a few minutes, you could identify quite a few people in your life that have been diagnosed with these diseases and disorders. It's just that widespread.

The following is a list and explanation of six common digestive afflictions, most of which have presented themselves in my own family. Maybe you will identify with one or more of them, or have already been diagnosed as having one. Please keep in mind that this is how prevalent digestive disease is. I personally have nine family members (out of twenty-two) who have been formally diagnosed with one or more of these diseases.

Irritable Bowel Syndrome

Irritable bowel syndrome (IBS) is a bowel disorder that is usually characterized by chronic abdominal pain, bloating, gas, and generally inconsistent bowel habits. Unfortunately for sufferers, IBS has no single, concrete cause, but we do have some pretty good clues into what might ignite this intestinal fight. Some ideas include brain-to-gut signal problems, GI motor issues, intestinal hypersensitivity, mental health problems (this one I'm not so thrilled with), bacterial infections and/or overgrowth, chemical imbalances, food sensitivity, and genetic predisposition.[15]

Because lactose intolerance and IBS have such similar symptoms,[16] a trial of a lactose-free diet should probably be recommended by your doctor. If your doctor has not recommended ditching the dairy, and your symptoms have not gotten better, I completely recommend just going ahead and doing this yourself. It won't hurt you at all to do your own investigation and eliminate dairy. An IBS diagnosis has also been commonly given to patients who eventually discover that they are hosting various pathogens, and/or parasites. If you think that you may have IBS, ask your doctor to be tested for these things, as well as lactose intolerance and celiac disease, in order to rule them out first. This move could save you a lot of time and unnecessary gut ache.

With IBS, diarrhea or constipation may predominate, or they may alternate, and are classified as IBS-D (diarrhea), IBS-C (constipation), IBS-M (mixed), or IBS-U (un-subtyped).[17] I would be an example of someone who had IBS-C. The diagnosis of IBS is one of exclusion, but the symptoms alone are generally pretty tell-tale, especially when other possibilities are ruled out.

Interestingly, there seems to be a consensus about a few different situations in which sufferers can look back on and recall their symptoms correlating with. These include a stressful life event, (personally, I can definitely trace the commencement of my IBS back to a not-so-hot relationship) a bowel infection or parasite, or the onset of adolescence. People suffering from IBS are more likely to also have acid reflux, chronic fatigue syndrome, fibromyalgia, headaches, and backaches.[18]

Although there is no cure for IBS, there are treatments that attempt to relieve symptoms, including recommended dietary adjustments and surgery.[19] IBS has no effect on life expectancy, but it is definitely a source of chronic, constant pain, fatigue, and other symptoms. This is a fabulous reason to change your diet and get better holistically. Mother Nature's remedies are free and fabulous! Here are some startling facts about IBS, the first three of which were taken directly from The National Digestive Diseases Information Clearinghouse (NDDIC):[20]

- "Up to twenty percent of the American population suffers from IBS.
- IBS affects almost twice as many women as men.
- IBS is most often diagnosed in people under the age of forty-five."[21]

These last four statistics are from the Canadian Digestive Health Foundation (CDHF):[22]

- "Patients with IBS miss an average of thirteen work days a year. This represents an annual figure of $8 million of lost productivity.
- About 40% of IBS sufferers seek medical attention.
- Acute care inpatient costs for IBS are ranked as the fourth most expensive digestive disease in Canada.
- Obesity enhances the severity of IBS symptoms."[23]

People suffering from IBS usually respond well to whole, easy-to-digest foods. Foods that contain no chemicals and highly absorbable nutrients are key here. For this reason, I personally consume a lot of liquids. I blend or juice fruits and vegetables several times each day, because I now understand that my body needs a break from foods that are more difficult to process. Also, by eliminating highly processed and altered foods, you can lighten the toxin load that is so difficult for your gut to deal with.

Diverticular Disease

Diverticular disease is the result of having diverticulosis (the formation of small pouches the bulge outward in your intestinal wall), and diverticulitis (the abscesses and subsequent infections that result from it).[24]

There are usually no signs that an individual has diverticulosis, but symptoms associated with diverticulitis are lower-left side stomach pain, fever, and chills. Sufferers might also complain of diarrhea or nausea, while others might report constipation. The severity of symptoms is largely dependent on the extent of the likely infection and subsequent complications. Diverticulitis may get worse as the day goes on, beginning as small pains and/or diarrhea, and gradually developing into vomiting and more pain.[25]

The development of this disease is thought to be caused by (drumroll please!) chronic constipation. A lack of dietary fiber, particularly non-soluble fiber (such as whole grains), may contribute largely to individuals developing diverticular disease.[26]

"Americans spend $1,300,069.00 a day on laxatives."[27]

—Paul Chek, holistic health practitioner

In most cases of uncomplicated diverticulitis accompanied by moderate acute infection, the sufferer can rest at home, limiting food consumption to liquids and repairing their weak intestinal tract with antibiotics.[28]

However, recurring episodes or complications may require surgery. Emergency surgery is often inescapable for people whose intestine has ruptured, because a rupture of this nature almost certainly results

Side note: Mild cases of diverticulitis do not necessarily require treatment of antibiotics. Antibiotics are far too over-prescribed and are mostly unnecessary for mild infection. Antibiotics kill all bacteria in the gut, even friendly bacteria. Without the friendly stuff, the cycle keeps perpetuating. Under the advice of a doctor, sufferers should make sure that their diverticulitis flare-up warrants the use of antibiotics, and try to use preventative measures with this disease instead of post-flare-up medications.

in an infected abdominal cavity.[29] During surgery, a colon-resection may be performed.[30]

Diverticulitis most often affects middle-aged and elderly persons, though it can strike young people too. Obesity is associated with diverticulitis in young patients, with some being as young as in their early twenties.[31] Usually, this goes back to the chronic constipation issue. Colon health is key here, folks. A dirty colon can contribute to all sorts of illness. Here are some stats from the World Gastroenterology Organisation[32] about diverticular disease:

- "2–5% of diverticular disease cases affect those under the age of forty.
- Between 22–30% of first-time patients will go on to have subsequent diverticular episodes.
- 30% of diverticular patients also have been diagnosed with IBS.
- Diverticular disease is less common among vegetarians."[33]

Here are some more facts from The Canadian Digestive Health Foundation[34]:

- "More than 130,000 Canadians have diverticular disease.
- Each year, 13,000 Canadians are admitted to hospitals due to the disease.
- Direct costs associated with diverticular disease are $88.6 million per year.
- The management of diverticular disease costs Canadians $90.3 million each year.
- 50% of Canadians over the age of eighty develop the disease.
- Diverticular disease is the fifth most expensive digestive disease to manage.
- Every year, more than 400 Canadians die due to complications associated with diverticular disease."[35]

Although not completely proven, it is often recommended that diverticulitis sufferers benefit from the absence of small foods that can easily become lodged in the inflamed pouches of their intestine. Foods such as seeds, nuts, and corn kernels fall into this category. Like IBS sufferers, those experiencing diverticulitis should also consider adopting a semi-liquid diet. To repair and restore a damaged intestinal wall, there needs to be the right type of nutrition being absorbed to help this process.

This is attainable by ditching the crap (literally), and introducing liquid nourishment in the form of blended or juiced organic fruits and veggies.

Inflammatory Bowel Disease

Contrary to IBS and diverticulitis, inflammatory bowel disease (IBD) is a completely different ball game. It consists of two major, closely related disorders, though each have their own unique twists. The first is colitis, and the second is Crohn's disease. I have two very good friends who are sisters, whom I have known for over ten years. One has colitis, and the other has Crohn's. I can tell you from my experiences with these two women that IBD is extremely debilitating, and results in the use of tremendous amounts of drugs and hospitalizations. It affects not only the body, but also the mind. It messes with self-esteem, and eventually takes on an all-encompassing and defining role in one's life. IBD is terrible, but it can be treatable, and probably in some cases preventable, too.

Colitis (sometimes it's ulcerative), affects the large bowel or colon. Inflammation can be acute or chronic, and the area is usually home to bleeding ulcers. People who live with chronic colitis symptoms are at a much greater risk for colon cancer than the general population.[36] This is due to the chronically aggravated condition of the colon.

Crohn's disease can occur anywhere within the intestinal tract, but is most common in the ileum or large bowel.[37] Crohn's disease typically has different symptoms than colitis, because of the variation of location. However, both diseases are painful, frightening, and exhausting. The following are statistics taken from The Crohn's and Colitis Foundation of America (CCFA):[38]

- "As many as 700,000 Americans suffer from Crohn's disease.
- Men and women are equally affected.
- Crohn's is most common among young adults, ranging in age from 15-35 years old.
- 5-20% of people who have been diagnosed with Crohn's have a first-degree relative with IBD.[39]
- Most people diagnosed with colitis are in their mid-thirties."[40]

Here are some more facts about inflammatory bowel disease from The Canadian Digestive Health Foundation:

- "In 2008, there were an estimated 250,000 Canadians with IBD.
- The total direct and indirect costs of IBD are $1.8 billion. The total direct medical costs for IBD were $700 million in 2008. In 2008, the cost of prescription drugs for the treatment of Canadian patients with IBD was $162 million. ($809 per patient). Costs associated with additional physician visits and outpatient surgeries were $134 million in 2008.
- Indirect costs associated with IBD total more than $1 billion with the main contributor being long-term work loss. Sick leave and absenteeism attributes to IBD cost the Canadian economy $104.2 million per year. Absenteeism and early retirement due to IBD is estimated to cost the Canadian market $746 million. In a single year, the Canadian workforce suffers a productivity loss of $138 million due to short-term absences of IBD patients.

- The average age of IBD onset coincides with an individual's most important socioeconomic period of their life. As such, the indirect costs of IBD are enormous as symptom severity may prevent a patient from realizing their career potential or family creation.
- Almost half of IBD patients have additional health issues affecting their joints, skin, eyes, and biliary tract that may be more debilitating than the bowel symptoms."[41]

Those living with IBD are in dire need of a nutritional overhaul. First and foremost, the intestines need repairing, stat. That means going on an elimination diet, where all animal products are omitted, as well as chemicals, processed foods, non-organics, and anything genetically modified. Although the liquid diet in the previous two sections can also be helpful for IBD, it is not recommended right away. Often, it will only aggravate diarrheal circumstances associated with a severely dysfunctional bowel.

Because of this, those with IBD should begin by consuming only foods that will not anger their digestive system. This usually entails forgoing any food with insoluble fiber, such as raw fruits and vegetables. Examples of produce that is easier to digest properly, are steamed or baked vegetables and starches, such as yams, sweet potatoes, apples, pears, carrots, beets, etc. Fruits and veggies are very important here, but they need to be slightly cooked in order to be more easily digestible. Also, the BRAT diet of bananas, brown, sprouted rice, applesauce, and whole grain, sprouted toast is recommended for those suffering from chronic diarrhea.[42] Daily digestive enzymes in the form of capsules can also be important, as well as probiotics, also available in capsule form. Lots of herbal teas and room temperature water are necessary to counter the loose bowel movements. Juicing is a really great way for people suffering from IBD to obtain vitamins and living enzymes from raw fruits and veggies. Because juicing removes the fiber, the liquid is generally tolerated much easier than the whole form is.[43] For more detailed instructions on a food plan tailored specifically for IBD, please consult a naturopath or plant-based dietician.

Celiac Disease

Celiac disease is an autoimmune disorder of the small intestine that occurs in people of all ages. Symptoms can include chronic diarrhea, failure to thrive (in children), rapid weight loss, and chronic fatigue.[44] In the United States population, nearly one out of every one hundred people is thought to have celiac disease.[45] It is caused by a reaction to gluten protein found in wheat, and similar proteins such as barley and rye. Upon exposure to the proteins in these grains, an inflammatory reaction occurs. This leads to damage of the villi lining of the small intestine which, in turn, interferes with the absorption of nutrients, because the intestinal villi are responsible for absorption.

The only known effective treatment for celiac disease is a long-term, gluten-free diet.

While the disease is caused by a reaction to wheat proteins, it is important to note that it is not the same as wheat allergy. It is easy to see why, in this situation, diet can literally mean life or death.

As the bowel becomes more damaged, lactose intolerance may develop. Often, sufferers are diagnosed with IBS and then, after more extensive testing, are found to actually have celiac disease. Blood tests are often prescribed first to make a diagnosis of celiac disease, and are typically followed up by a biopsy of the duodenum.[46] This disease is serious. Celiac disease leads to an increased risk of colorectal cancer if left untreated, and may lead to other complications, eventually resulting in death. Here are some facts about celiac disease from the National Foundation for Celiac Awareness:[47]

- "More than 3 million Americans have celiac disease.
- About 85% of Americans who have this disease are undiagnosed.

- 5–22% of patients diagnosed with celiac disease have an immediate family member who also has it."[48]

Here are more stats and facts from the Canadian Digestive Health Foundation:

- "More than 330,000 Canadians have been diagnosed with celiac disease. More than 73,000 are children.
- Nearly 30% of Canadian children with celiac disease are initially misdiagnosed.
- 30% of celiac patients may develop a malignancy (non-Hodgkin's lymphoma) if left untreated."[49]

The cure for celiac disease? A gluten-free diet. That's it! This is amazing and important knowledge. If you think you might have this disorder, please go get tested. It could save your life.

Gastroesophageal Reflux Disease (GERD)

Acid reflux is a chronic symptom of mucosal damage caused by stomach acid or bile coming up from the stomach into the esophagus. When this process occurs several times a week, and/or begins to affect your daily life, it is called gastroesophageal reflux disease, or GERD.[50]

The most common adult symptoms of GERD are mild-severe heartburn, regurgitation, and trouble swallowing.[51] Here are two statistics from *American Family Physician:*[52]

- 10% of Americans experience heartburn every day.
- GERD affects approximately 25–35% of the American population. [53]

Here are some more stats from The Canadian Digestive Health Foundation:

- On average, five million Canadians experience heartburn and/or acid regurgitation at least once each week.

- 42% of GERD patients are dissatisfied with the outcome of drug therapy.
- GERD patients are absent from work 16% of each year due to their symptoms. In Canada, this represents a workforce productivity loss of 1.7 billion hours amounting to $21 billion each year. Yikes!
- Increasing age is recognized as a primary risk factor for the development of GERD.[54]

Dietary changes are recommended, such as consuming a diet low in acidity and richness, including (plug for plant-based diet!) no red meat, dairy, alcohol, or overly acidic fruits or vegetables. Caffeine, peppermint, and anything tomato-based seems to be difficult to tolerate. Also, it is recommended that sufferers sleep on their side.

Lactose Intolerance & Casein Allergies

This last affliction is so incredibly common, and many people experience these symptoms without ever knowing that dairy is the culprit. In fact, as you have already read, celiac disease, lactose intolerance, and casein allergies can all be (and all have been) mistaken for IBS.

Let's just face it: we are all somewhat intolerant to milk, particularly cow's milk. In fact, it's the lactose (cows' milk sugar) and the casein (cows' milk protein) with which we, as human beings, have a tough time. And why shouldn't we? We are drinking another animal's milk! It is not made for us to digest properly; it is meant for fattening up baby calves. It contains way more fat than humans could ever need, because cows get big. (As in approximately ten times the weight of adult humans.) If calves were fed human breast milk, they'd probably die of starvation! We don't even drink our own milk, past the age of a year or two. Furthermore, the two types of milk are hardly comparable. Human milk is perfectly created for humans, with just the right amount of protein, carbohydrates, sugars, and other nutrients. Everything in it is easily digestible and relatively low in fat, because most of us don't reach a healthy adult weight of more than 110–180 pounds. Adult cows, however, generally end up anywhere between 1100 and 2500 pounds, and so definitely need more protein, more carbohydrates, and a ton of fat. It's perfect for *them*. No other species shares its milk with another, except maybe in extreme cases, where an orphaned puppy has nursed from a new mother pig. (I know I've seen something like that on YouTube.)

Lactose is the sugar in dairy products. Those who are lactose intolerant lack the enzyme (lactase) to break down this sugar for proper absorption. When the lactose reaches the large bowel (colon), it causes gas, bloating, diarrhea and abdominal cramping.[55] Here is some more information about this crazy common affliction from Ohio State University:

- "30–50 million Americans are lactose intolerant.
- Lactose is used as the main ingredient in over 20% of prescription medication. (Including, ironically, meds for acid reflux and gas.)
- Symptoms most commonly begin 30 minutes to 2 hours after consuming foods with lactose."[56]
- Here are some more facts about lactose intolerance from The Canadian Digestive Health Foundation:
- "Lactose intolerance affects more than seven million Canadians. This is likely an underestimate as many individuals do not associate their symptoms with lactose-containing foods or are asymptomatic.
- Since only 10% of symptomatic patients are clinically tested (294,000 people), it appears that Canadian physicians underestimate the daily impact of chronic lactose intolerant symptoms.
- 25% of patients clinically identified as lactose intolerant have celiac disease. In Canada, that means that 73,500 people

have undiagnosed celiac disease, which is the causal agent for their lactose intolerance.

- A digestive disease patient may consume ten grams or more of lactose each day from their (prescription) drugs."[57] Seems a little counter-productive, doesn't it?

The treatment? Stop consuming dairy. It's that simple. Easy peasy, lemon squeezy! More information on most of these diseases can be found at the National Digestive Diseases Information Clearinghouse (http://digestive.niddk.nih.gov/index.aspx) or at www.ibsgroup. org. The latter website also offers forums in which IBS and other intestinal disorder sufferers can sign up and lend support to each other. These web links are also listed in the Resources section, at the end of the book.

Question: Have you been tested for any of the above digestive disorders? Do you think one of them sounds like what you may be experiencing? Talk to your doctor, but don't go to your appointment empty-handed. Keep a food journal. Write down specific symptoms. If you know a certain food bothers you, such as wheat or dairy, make a note of that. The more information you can provide your doctor with, the better he or she can help you. Take care of this now, or it will get worse. If the idea of seeing a doctor just throws you off your game, then inquire about obtaining an appointment with a local naturopath, or a registered holistic nutritionist.

Highlight: Judy's Story

How is it that we can often become so desensitised to discomfort and exhaustion? I wonder if, for many women, it starts when we have our babies, and then just never leaves us entirely. I think when I was younger, in my teens and later before pregnancy, I had such a high metabolism that I didn't notice that not being "regular" made me feel unwell. Much to my daughter's dismay, a constant saying in my life has been "my guts ache."

When I became pregnant, I was used to being bloated and tired. When I had newborns, I was exhausted, and finding time to sit down and actually eat an entire meal was a hit or miss opportunity at best. By the time my children were toddlers, I had adjusted to the reality of iffy energy and had started my journey into the land of chronic headaches, constipation, and gut aches. And I thought this was all pretty normal. Don't all women go through these phases?

Around the age of thirty, I once had such severe abdominal pain that my hands and feet went completely numb. It was incredibly frightening, and my husband called an ambulance for me. I was taken to the emergency room at the local hospital and checked out. The attending physician told me that I had experienced a flair-up of irritable bowel syndrome, and that the pain had made me breathe very shallowly, which in turn had caused the numbness in my extremities. I was sent home with no other information.

Okay. IBS. It was just another gut ache.

Then, by the time my children were teenagers, the gut aches intensified and became a daily event for about eighteen months. During this time, there were several occasions where I found myself sitting on the toilet in extreme pain. It literally felt like I was labouring in childbirth. I imagined having a prolapsed intestine . . .

Around the same time period, my daughter came home a couple of times and told me she couldn't eat anything that used to have a face. This stopped me cold. How could I eat anything that used to have a face?! (This reminded me of the time when I was small and learned that an egg was the "big cell." I came home and told my mom I couldn't eat "the big cell." And I didn't for a few years . . . and then like we all do, I found a way to ignore where meat and eggs come from. I preferred to think of all the meat in the grocery store beginning and ending in that little cellophane wrapped package in the cooler. If I didn't think about it, it wouldn't bother me.) So, we all started dabbling in eating vegetarian fare. We would eat a couple of plant-based meals a week, but most of my meals still had meat, poultry and fish, and I still had lots of cheese and creams.

And my guts still hurt.

This just became the norm, along with being bloated and having frequent headaches, right through my forties and into my fifties. Then, one day when I was driving home from a lunch out with girlfriends, my stomach really started to hurt way more than ever before. It took about an hour to get home from that lunch, and by the time I arrived back to my community, I knew I had to go straight to the hospital. After a CT scan, I got a diverticulitis diagnosis, and spent the next five days in the hospital; four of them in a bed in a hallway. That was just over a year ago, and I have been struggling with diverticulitis symptoms ever since. The biggest challenges are getting enough fiber, having daily bowel movements, and being hydrated enough. Constipation is deadly, and I have been living a lifetime with chronic constipation.

After watching my daughter switch to a vegetarian diet and seeing her progress and immense improvement, I decided to give it a try too. I was a little bit worried about not fitting in with the others at the dinner table, or becoming a problem at home. My spouse is not a vegetarian, but not only does he not care that I have given up meat, he completely supports me. He makes me well balanced dinners when I come home from work, and is always researching new recipes to use for me. My refrigerator is often stocked up with a wide variety of vegetables, fruit and nuts from his shopping trips.

If you are going to adopt a plant-based diet, I want to inform you about week one, as my daughter did for me. The first week I was meat free, I had low to no energy and several headaches, and for the first few days, my constipation continued. My insides were so, so bloated and my bowels were in shock. By the end of the first week, I felt more energetic and the headaches stopped and the bowel movements became so amazing, that they would make Dr. Oz proud! So stay focused and expect some symptoms of detoxification for a few days. You are ridding your body of a substance that has been clogging it up for your entire life. You will get past it, and reap huge rewards almost overnight. If you have a digestion issue, whether it be one of the diseases that is discussed in this book, or something entirely different that you feel will benefit from the absence of meat, do this. Eat whole and plant-based foods. As long as I stay on the wagon, eating a plant-based diet gives me my life back, and for the first time in decades, I can honestly say that I feel great. My guts no longer ache.

Chapter 4

Inflammation Nation

"Less elastic skin, arthritis, poorer memory, and even heart conditions are often attributable to inflamed tissue."[58]
—Brendan Brazier, *The Thrive Diet*

It has been said that at the root of every chronic disease lies inflammation. Inflammation is caused by our white blood cells attacking problem areas when we hurt ourselves, are battling viruses, or when the body identifies something foreign that needs to be addressed. When we are constantly feeding ourselves inflammatory foods, which our body rightly recognizes as a problem, this reaction becomes the norm. After a certain period of time, chronic inflammation leads to diseases, such as diabetes, heart disease, digestive diseases, colon cancer (often attributed to chronic inflammation of the colon), arthritis, asthma, and Alzheimer's disease.[59] In order to try and reduce your chances of developing one of these diseases, or to treat a current disease of this nature, you must get rid of anything that might be contributing to unnecessary inflammation.

What Chronic Inflammation Means to You

A good example of purposeful inflammation reduction is the elimination of dairy from the diet of someone experiencing asthmatic and/or seasonal allergy symptoms, as well as those suffering from chronic ear infections. Numerous studies have shown that by eradicating dairy (which is very inflammatory) from their diets, people can lessen their symptoms of these chronic medical nuisances, or even completely ditch them altogether.[60] In fact, it is common practice for a pediatrician who deals with childhood allergies and ear infections to recommend that the child cease to consume dairy completely. In my case, I know that about thirty minutes to two hours after consuming dairy, my stomach will begin to bloat and cramp. Bloating is a symptom of inflammation. The following lists are my go-to foods and my cease-and-destroy ones:

Foods that Reduce Inflammation

1. Vegetables. Raw veggies are full of living enzymes that your gut adores. Your tummy goes all drooly and ga-ga for raw veggies. Feed the beast!

2. Water. Water is key to reducing inflammation. What's the first thing you want to do in the height of summer, after spending all day outside getting red and swollen? Take a cold shower! If you can see the anti-inflammatory results from water on the outside, imagine what is happening when you drink it on the inside. Water equals awesomeness!

3. Spices. Spices like ginger, turmeric, and cinnamon are naturally anti-inflammatory foods. They have strong flavors to entice us to ingest them, so get on it!

4. Omega-3s. Anything containing naturally high levels of this essential fatty acid, such as nuts, nut butters, algae, seeds, olives, and avocados, is key to good health. This is really great news for me, because I love olives! (Especially when they're stuffed with garlic.) On a western diet, we get way too many

omega 6 fatty acids. This creates an uneven fatty acid ratio, which ideally should be 1:1. Eating more omega-3s will help to regain this ratio, and so will eating foods in their whole form.

5. Green tea. This oldie but goodie is known for its anti-inflammatory properties and antioxidant loveliness. Drink up some green love!

Foods that Inflame

The following foods are a western diet junkie's dream, but are very bad for causing inflammation:

1. Sugar. This highly addictive substance is the number one inflammatory food. It's bad, and the more refined, the worse it makes you feel. If you don't believe me, try eliminating all sugar from your diet for two weeks. I'll bet you get super grumpy, lethargic, and headachy throughout the duration of week one. In your second week you will feel great. Then, when you board the crazy sugar train again at the end of the fourteen days, you will really experience sugar's wrath. It's addictive, manipulative, and messes with your body from the inside out. Blech!

2. Alcohol. (One of the reasons people look so puffy after a bender, along with fluid retention.) Alcohol breaks down into pure sugar, so just go ahead and read the sugar rant again.

3. Refined grains. White rice, white bread, and white pasta are just more examples of highly refined, crappy sugar.

4. Dairy products. Because dairy was never meant to be consumed by humans, but we all seem to think it's a health food and consume a lot of it, it really has its way with us. Like sugar, it's addictive. Why? Because it has a lot of sugar in it! ("*ose*" at the end of a word indicates sugar, like fructose, glucose, sucrose and, you guessed it, lactose!)

5. Trans-fats. These are found in foods such as margarine and fast food. Trans-fats are weird. They are a liquid-turned-solid that never really break down and are completely preserved and last forever on the floor of your garage. True story.

These foods are not only incredibly inflammatory; they are also devoid of nutrients. There is no point to eat them ever. They should be moved to your naughty list, stat. By eating the foods in the first list, and skipping the foods on the last list, you will be able to feel an almost immediate transformation within your newly, cooled-off body. Within a week, you will look and feel less bloated, retain less water, your eyes will appear less puffy, and you will probably lose a few pounds, too. Yippee!

General Food Sensitivities

Nowadays, you'd be hard-pressed to find someone who doesn't live with some sort of food sensitivity. I say "nowadays" because I, along with many others, genuinely believe that this problem was not as prevalent in the past as it is today.[61] With the way we currently process food, and routinely add chemical cocktails to enhance it for the ultimate purpose of generating more money, food sensitivities are now inevitable. I almost guarantee that you have heard someone from the baby-boomer generation comment that "no one was allergic to peanuts in *my* day." I'm not saying that nut allergies are new, but they are definitely more mainstream. So are wheat, gluten, dairy, seafood, corn, and soy. And egg. And food coloring. And . . .

Let me explain. Because of the western world's incredible obsession with convenience, we have inevitably begun to eat some of the same foods several times a day in ways we are often unaware of. We are constantly inundated with wheat, corn, soy, sugar, salt, and casein products, as well as a wide variety of chemicals such as MSG (monosodium glutamate), food coloring, and artificial flavoring. These ingredients are present in almost everything processed, and because we consume so much of them, and they come to us in such overly processed forms, our digestive system eventually decides that it has had enough, and so challenges our immune system to a duel. En garde!

This is especially true for those of us who already have a slight sensitivity to one or more of these ingredients. We can only expect our digestive systems to take on so much, and after that, we feel the refusal. For example, I can abstain from cheese for a month and feel great, and I can eat a little bit here and there without feeling the negative effects, but if I decide one night to chow down on an entire wheel of brie with my beloved olives (something that I have unfortunately done *several* times), I always pay for it. It's like my body grudgingly will process bit by bit until I overdo it, and then it shuts down and becomes terribly inflamed. I always regret it.

Cheese is my boyfriend that I know is bad for me in every single way, but I keep coming back for more despite the very predictable consequences. If I had a cheese therapist, she would tell me to break the cycle. You break it, too!

"Let food be thy medicine and thy medicine be thy food."[62]
—Hippocrates, father of modern medicine

So many of us are living with food sensitivities like this and don't know it; it's hard to make the connection when pain is unpredictable and sometimes random. I personally only discovered my dairy issue when I cut out meat. Because the heaviness of meat was out of the picture, and my inflammation was greatly reduced, I was able to feel the other foods that made me feel bad, too. Wheat, dairy, and meat all make me feel swollen, bloated, and in pain. It sounds like a lot that I've had to remove from my life, but the difference in how I feel can only be described as amazing, and for me, it's undeniably worth it. I also welcome other fabulous side-effects of this diet, such as being able to stay at my desired weight effortlessly. For me, it's just not worth it to eat the foods that make me feel bad. I love feeling good, and I sure as hell love feeling good in a bathing suit!

Besides the ones previously listed, foods high in acidity, such as tomatoes and animal meat, can trigger a sensitivity-like effect. In addition, food additives, such as artificial colors, flavors, nitrates, and MSG can cause small reactions that you may not even be aware of. Take note of what makes you feel badly, log it in your "foods-that-make-me-feel-like-shit" book, and try eliminating it for awhile. See how you feel. Reintroduce it and notice if it has an effect on you. You can also get an allergy/sensitivity test done by a local naturopath.

Chronic inflammation is scary. It means that your body is overreacting to something that is bothering it on a consistent basis. It should be a warning sign to you if any part of your body is always inflamed. For me, and many other digestive disorder sufferers, inflamed intestines are a very real deal. IBD, IBS, lactose intolerance, and diverticulitis, in particular, are extremely inflammatory disorders. If you suffer from one of these, I urge you to help your body. Eat foods that fight inflammation, not the ones that cause or provoke it. Try the garlic-stuffed olives . . .

Question: Do you have noticeable bloating after eating a meal? Bloating is a sign of inflammation, and you can only feel and see a small percentage of what is actually occurring in your body. If you notice that you bloat after eating certain foods, then stop eating them! Your body is trying to show you what's happening; let it know you're paying attention.

Chapter 5

Healthcare 9-1-1

" . . . the factory farm industry (in alliance with the pharmaceutical industry) currently has more power than public-health professionals. We give it to them. We have chosen, unwittingly, to fund this industry on a massive scale by eating factory-farmed animal products . . . and we do so daily."[63]

—Jonathan Safran Foer, *Eating Animals*

Obvious to many, something is happening that is changing the quality of our health. These changes might seem small or relative to the general population, but they aren't. More people are dying from chronic yet preventable diseases than ever before. People are getting sicker faster and younger. Despite taking into account the population increase within the last one hundred years, diseases, such as diabetes, heart disease, cancers, hypertension, chronic and debilitating digestive ailments, and obesity are on the rise like never seen before, and I mean never.[64] So, what the hell is going on? One word: nutrition. Or rather, lack thereof . . .

We are in the middle of a healthcare crisis of epidemic (soon to be pandemic)proportions in Canada and the United States. There are two major factors that are responsible for this, in my opinion.

The first is our affinity for the western diet, which is certainly the norm in these two countries, and unfortunately, is quickly becoming quite popular everywhere else in the world, too. The western diet comprises foods that are mostly . . . well, not really food.

Fast food, processed food, factory-farmed animal products, and a slew of chemicals including preservatives, stabilizers, artificial coloring and flavors, pesticides, genetically modified organisms and more, make up the bulk of the average North American's diet. This diet is unprecedented in not only its laboratory-created component, but also in the effects it has had, and rapidly continues to have, on our swiftly declining, collective health.

The second factor contributing to our healthcare despair is our medical professionals' inability to deal with this problem, because of their lack of proper nutrition education, and abundance of opportunistic misinformation from the meat, dairy, and pharmaceutical industries that are incredibly effective in convincing our doctors to push their products. (You'd be hard-pressed to find a North American general practitioner who would tell you that milk isn't good for you. It "does a body good"[65] doesn't it?)

Factory-farmed animal products are just one example of how we are causing detriment to our health, typically without us knowing so. Misguided information and general ignorance towards what is being put in our food is literally killing us. American general practitioners have an average of twenty hours' worth of nutrition education, with eighteen of those hours being centered on infant formula.[66] This means that a nutritionist, who possesses considerably less education than a medical doctor (typically one to two years of study compared to ten to twelve), has more basic knowledge about diet and nutrition than a heart surgeon who deals with the effects of coronary heart disease, contracted in most part by terrible dietary choices that often occur on a daily basis.

This is a major problem.

In fact, as Dr. T. Colin Campbell emphasizes in *The China Study*, which is a thirty-eight year-long study that shows a very strong correlation between cascin (cow milk protein) and cancer, "the health damage that results from doctors' ignorance of nutrition is astounding."[67]

When confronted with treating patients who have any type of chronic disease (not limited to digestive disease), most doctors will order expensive tests, prescribe expensive drugs, and if all else fails, recommend expensive surgeries. All of this expense adds up to an unbelievable sum of money spent on treatments that are typically ineffective, or could be treated more efficiently through dietary changes and real, fact-based, nutrition education for the public. Ergo, our skyrocketing healthcare costs and devastating, life-threatening cuts. Who benefits from dealing with our health issues in this typically ineffective and overly expensive manner?

Pharmaceutical companies do.

If you were able to eradicate your digestive disease symptoms naturally, it would amount to billions of dollars in lost drug sales for major drug companies. It's deeply unfortunate, but it is not in anyone's interest but your own to actually cure what ails you. That means that only *you* can accomplish this properly, through food and lifestyle rehabilitation. Don't take that as scary or hopeless information . . . it's some damn empowering knowledge! Use it to your advantage, mon ami!

An example of this inefficiency to unearth the root of digestion problems in order to heal from the bottom up is the story of my friend Kim, who is one of the sisters I mentioned in chapter three, in the section on IBD (page 23). Kim was diagnosed with Crohn's disease at the age of nineteen, although she says she can remember digestive malfunction occurring as early as seven years old.

When, at the age of twenty-seven, she could no longer cope, she underwent two and a half weeks of testing that included a barium enema, a CT-scan, and numerous x-rays. After pondering the results of these examinations, Kim's doctors gave her an ultimatum: she could either begin steroids which would have cost her hundreds of dollars per injection, or she could have major stomach surgery, where they would ultimately perform a resection of her bowel. So, because Kim could not afford such an expensive alternative, she had a one foot-long damaged portion of her small intestine removed, along with a six-inch section of her colon. This left her with a crude scar that is about seven inches long, running from her navel to her hip bone, and she was kept in the hospital for over three weeks to recover.

During her recovery, her doctors administered the steroids that she had refused up until this point without her permission. She felt no physical (and certainly no psychological) relief from the surgery or the steroids, and regretted it within months. In fact, because of her scar, she has since become self-conscious, too. The hospital staff also administered morphine and ciprofloxacin to Kim, even though she was wearing a medical bracelet stating her allergy to these medications, as well as the information being clearly included in her chart. After these events, her doctor tried to persuade her to begin more steroids that would, in theory, put her Crohn's into remission. She refused, believing there must be a better way to manage the symptoms, without having to experience the numerous side-effects of the steroid. Up until this point, she had gotten by with regular prescriptions of antibiotics to manage the inevitable, constant, and recurrent kidney infections that are associated with her condition.

Kim was told nothing about what to expect with the surgery or the subsequent pain and recovery. She was given no information about proper nutrition for a Crohn's patient, let alone what foods she should eat or avoid eating right after having the surgery. The parting communication that she had with her doctor was him trying to convince her to fill a prescription for the pain killer Demerol. She didn't. Her Crohn's symptoms were back within two months after the reassurance of her doctors that she should experience one to twenty years of relief from the surgery.

At twenty-nine, she began a more natural process of managing her health that seemed to work, at least temporarily. Her regimen included daily doses of slippery elm, white willow, aloe vera capsules, oil of oregano, iron, and vitamin B12. She gave up alcohol, and started to pay more attention to her diet. This lifestyle change worked better than anything she had tried before, and the effects lasted for about a year before her chronic symptoms came back, coinciding with a series of stressful situations.

As I write this sentence, at the age of thirty-one, she is debating those steroids.

She is always exhausted, because she averages about two hours of sleep per night due to her inability to rest properly, something that is also symptomatic of Crohn's. She is always in pain, which has led to chronic stress and low self-esteem. Among other ideas, she has recently had a specialist make the ludicrous suggestion that she eat only processed baby food! She is completely confused, and at a loss for inspiration. Recently, Kim discovered that she was approved for a new type of drug, administered via bi-weekly injections. This "miracle" medication will cost her $1200 per injection, unless she can get a government subsidy for it. That's $2400 a month, more than double her monthly mortgage payment.

Kim's doctors have never suggested she follow a restricted diet plan, rich in quality nutrients. She has met with numerous specialists over the years, and none of them have ever recommended making a lifestyle change that included stress-relief strategies, dietary improvements, exercise, or anything else that could help her without painkillers, steroids, or major surgical interventions. Drugs and surgery are all she can ever remember being discussed. She even admits that when she brings up the possibility of a more holistic treatment, her doctors become dismissive and even angry with her.

Why is the obvious question of food quality often left out of the initial diagnosis when it comes to digestive disorders? It's confusing, and, unfortunately for those suffering, it's the norm.

The situation with Kim has left us both feeling that there is something incredibly wrong with our current healthcare system. In a structural scheme where surgeries and medications come before common sense and dietary intervention, and where the average general practitioner in the United States completes only about two credits worth of nutritional training in their entire university career,[68] what do we have to lose by taking our precious health into our own hands, and begin walking a road of healing by simply altering our own eating habits?

When we can't fathom food as being something that directly affects or has the power to change our digestive health, what does that say about our relationship with it? When did food get put on the backburner as the answer to digestive health, never mind health in general? Why are we so relentlessly obsessed with turning to medications, whose results are typically menial at best, and whose side effects generally greatly outweigh any possible benefits or relief?

A Quick Fix?

We live in a world that is sympathetic to our vices, and offers help in the form of a veil. We are significantly sicker now than ever before. We seem to have lost alot of what originally got us here to begin with. Lives used to be lived for our families, our happiness, good friends, and good food. What words do you associate with these ideals?

I'll bet the average American, without even knowing it, thinks of an Applebee's commercial when supplied with these images.

We need to get back to close families, outdoor recreation, breathing deep, slowing down, and eating fresh food that is even a little bit supplied by ourselves. It's sometimes hard to remember that the correct answer is most often the obvious one. Need to lose weight? Eat less, eat better food, and exercise more. Want better quality family time? Hang out together, play together, and talk amongst yourselves. Need to reconnect with old friends? Invite them over for a meal, laugh, and share your life a little. Everyone is looking for extra hours in the day, but how many hours do we spend in front of the television, on the phone, or staring at our laptops? By changing your food, you can change your life. You can ease digestion, encourage weight loss, aid elimination, reduce stress, and get back to Earth.

As in, "Earth to Jen! Are you there, Jen?"

I have been completely guilty of using every single one of the following bandage solutions in the past, but not anymore. Happily, I got back to Earth. (Yay!) You can too. This next list is my old assembly of quick fixes:

1. Diet pills or shakes for weight loss
2. Laxatives & stool softeners to induce bowel movements
3. Various over-the-counter meds to halt diarrhea
4. Sleeping pills to fall and stay asleep
5. Various vitamin, mineral, and herbal supplements
6. Hemorrhoid cream to banish BFFs
7. Yeast infection medication to control sugary yeast issues in the nether-regions

All of these crutches can be completely eliminated by adopting a clean, whole, plant-based diet. They exist to mask symptoms and/or provide a temporary solution to a (usually) recurrent problem. None of these items are necessary to take for longer than a couple of days, and only in dire situations.Luckily, everything that they promise to solve for you, I guarantee that good, whole, thoughtful food can do significantly better. If you are going to eat the way that I outline later on in this book, you will never have a need for any of these things ever again. Food becomes your complete nourishment, and takes care of you in every single way. It's like being wrapped up in a warm blanket and rocked to sleep at night. You feel calm, happy, cozy, and in tune with your body. It's crazy and awesome, and it's about time.

The Winds of Change

"If Americans stopped overeating, stopped eating unhealthy foods, and instead ate more foods with higher nutrient densities and cancer-protective properties, we could have a more affordable, sustainable, and effective healthcare system."[69]
—John Robbins, *No Happy Cows*

Dr. Dean Ornish is the perfect example of how we have the power to change the conventional treatment of chronic disease. He is president and founder of the non-profit Preventive Medicine Research Institute in Sausalito, California, as well as Clinical Professor of Medicine at the University of California, San Francisco.[70] For more than thirty years, he has worked to systematically to prove that diet and lifestyle directly contribute to coronary heart disease, diabetes, obesity, hypertension, and other western diseases. His philosophy includes adopting a healthy, whole food, plant-based diet coupled with stress reducing activities, such as yoga and meditation. Not only has Dr. Ornish been able to prove his theories about reducing the above diseases through diet; he has also proven that you can reverse them. His plan is so successful that various medical insurance companies in the United States, including Medicare, have agreed to cover his patients.[71] Now that's some serious proof!

Not only is this amazing news for those of us looking for ways to genuinely improve our own health naturally, but it's also great news for our healthcare system. If we could all be prescribed this lifestyle change instead of the insane amount of drug prescriptions and surgeries, we could collectively save alot of money, and alot of tummy aches. I believe that an immense change in current medical philosophy and practice is forthcoming, but we could start healing now. Why wait for the average Joe? Why not heal ourselves, and then help Joe heal himself too?

Dr. Ornish is not the only one campaigning for better nutrition. Other well-known professionals in the field of health include Dr. Caldwell Esselstyn, author of *Prevent and Reverse Heart Disease*, who has been advocating a plant-based diet for almost thirty years, and Dr. T. Colin Campbell, co-author of *The China Study*. All three of these men live and breathe a healthy, whole food, vegetarian lifestyle, and all are in incredible health. Dr. Neal Barnard, author of *Foods That Heal*, is another famous American doctor who believes in the ability of plants to heal our aches and pains, and there are many, many more. No one else offers advice on how to prevent sickness, eradicate current disease, and improve quality of life in the same ways that these men do.

What do we have to lose, besides a few pounds and a sack full of prescription medication?

Why Adopting this Wellness Plan Works

Many of you are probably skeptical as to why a whole food, plant-based plan works wonders, while other plans will also claim that they can do the same thing, but fail. This plan works because it's not so much a diet plan; it's a life plan; a full-on lifestyle recalibration of your entire way of thinking about and consuming food. You are making an active decision to change your life, because pain, among other things, is motivating you to do so. Armed with this powerful way of considering your food and how consuming it will help or hinder you, you ultimately end up eating food that is real, genuine nourishment. Your body recognizes the food as nutrients, and processes them accordingly. Pure foods create a clean result, and you will feel it almost immediately. This works, especially where digestion is concerned. There is alot of information out there about how a whole food, plant-based diet can cure diabetes and heart disease, hypertension and obesity problems. Most digestive diseases won't kill you the way heart disease can, but they can certainly make your life a living hell.

In the book (and film documentary) *Forks Over Knives*, editor Gene Stone outlines on page five what many of the book's featured physicians consider to be the key principles of a whole food, plant-based diet, and I'd have to agree with them whole-heartedly:

1. "Eat plants. The more intact, the better." More intact, meaning less processed, less cooked, less messed with or altered. To receive the full benefits of plant foods (and they are countless), you should eat most of them raw, most of the time. Our bodies know exactly what to do with raw fruits and veggies, because they are small miracles of amazing digestion. Again, your tummy goes bonkers over these marvelous morsels!

2. "Avoid overly processed foods." Foods that are highly processed, including meat and dairy, are stripped of their original nutrients (meat through cooking; dairy through pasteurization), and can no longer help your digestion but, instead, will hinder it. There are too many added chemicals, and your body becomes overrun, tired, and confused.

3. "Avoid preservatives and additives." Again, these items obviously aren't good for you. They are added to food for the sole purpose of being able to extend the product's shelf life, which should be a warning sign right there. You don't want to be eating anything that lives longer than your pet goldfish; especially in room temperature! (Ummm . . . did someone say margarine?)

4. "Eliminate dairy." As a self-proclaimed dairy maniac, this one is sad, but so, so true. Dairy is not good for you, no matter how many milk posters you've seen. The dairy industry is a very lucrative one, and sadly, dairy is pushed for that reason

alone. Lactose intolerance is probably the leading cause of digestive distress.

5. "Don't worry about carbohydrates." Yay! Don't even try and tell me you're not excited at this prospect. The anti-carb movement has been around far too long, and again, people are only getting more and more sick. Making smart carbohydrate choices (complex carbohydrates in the form of whole, unprocessed or minimally processed grains) will give you much more long-lasting energy and help you lose weight, not make you gain. There is way too much false information about the role of carbs out there, and we are paying the price. Carbs are not the enemy!

6. "Don't worry about not getting enough protein." Again, I realize you're still in shock from the carbohydrate statement, but here it is again: don't stress about your protein intake. Newsflash: vegetables contain protein! (Don't fall over. In fact, maybe you should sit down.) We don't need animal products, or even protein powder to crank up our consumption of this nutrient. There is a huge misconception about how much protein we need to be healthy.[72] Have you ever heard of someone in the developed world having a protein deficiency? Probably not. If you are consuming enough calories to keep you healthy, then you are getting enough protein. Are you sitting as suggested, or passed out on the floor in disbelief? Well, this fact is true, folks, and very well documented.

7. "Don't worry about omega-3 fatty acids." The reason that people fret over omega 3's is because we've all been told that there needs to be a proper ratio (1:1-1:3) of omega 3's to omega 6's, and we eat far too many omega 6's. Therefore, we must eat more omega 3's. (I talked about their role in reducing inflammation in chapter four.) However, if we were all on a plant-centered, whole and healthy diet, that ratio would naturally fall into its proper proportions. Mother

Nature knows what to do—trust her. Don't manipulate or forget about her. Girls hate that.

8. "Consider a vitamin B12 supplement." I will talk more about this special nutrient later, but the gist is this: we used to get enough of this naturally, but by messing up the quality of our topsoil through recent, crazy agricultural practices (broad-spray fertilizer/pesticides, etc), we don't get it anymore by eating a plant-based diet. We are capable of obtaining enough of this vitamin by eating meat, because the animals have eaten enough of it via plants, and are passing it on to us. However, on a plant-based diet, you need to consider getting this nutrient in the form of a supplement.

Why this Lifestyle Modification Works

1. You stop poisoning yourself. Artificial chemicals, such as preservatives, colors, flavors, antibiotics, growth hormones and more, cease to infiltrate your body. And I haven't even touched on cosmetic chemicals yet! Prescription medications will eventually be rendered unnecessary, and your body will thank you for that too. (Consult a physician before going off any meds, though. It's easy to imagine why that might be a good idea ...)

2. You give your digestive system a break. Substances like the ones I just listed above are confusing for your body to deal with. Because of this confusion, your body deals with it in ways that create problems for you in the future. (For example, too much sugar intake contributing to a worn-out pancreas and the emergence of diabetes. Or, digestively speaking, too many animal products clogging up your colon and creating chronic disease there.)

3. You naturally detoxify your body and your intestines by sweeping out toxic debris that live there, through clean,

whole, plant-based eating. Brown, sprouted rice does a much better job of clearing the intestinal tract than polished, white rice does.

4. You allow your organs to clean up, and begin healing. This way, they can deal with their processes and do their specific jobs more efficiently. If your liver is constantly run down trying to filter out toxins that don't belong there, eventually it is going to give up. Hello, liver failure!

5. Your body needs energy to heal and repair. It also needs a certain amount of vitamins and minerals to help accomplish these tasks. By adopting a whole food, plant-based diet, you automatically meet every level of the vital nutrients needed. You will not be filling up on junk; you will be eating nourishing foods that will help you from the inside out. (Believe me; you will see it on the out, too!)

"Nutrition is critical for health. Many Americans are taking numerous medications three to four times a day, yet they haven't changed the dietary regimen that made them sick in the first place. Most people are not aware that these foods are, if anything, more powerful than the drugs."[73]

—Dr. Neal Barnard, *Forks Over Knives*

Question: Would you rather be prescribed medication, or be prescribed a lifestyle makeover, sans meds? One choice is the easy way, but it only masks the symptoms and doesn't actually solve the problem. In fact, it might exacerbate it, and it's a short-term solution at best. The second choice gets to the root of the issue, but requires education, persistence, and will power. However, this solution really is a solution; it's long-term. Hint: take option number two!

Highlight: Kelly's Story

I was diagnosed with colitis in 1994, when I was nineteen years old. Inflammatory bowel disease (IBD) runs in my family; my oldest sister and my mom also have colitis, and my youngest sister has Crohn's disease.

I had considered my colitis to be in remission for a long time (about thirteen years), when I began my most recent flare-up. This particular episode (which was pretty consistent with colitis symptoms), included major constipation alternating with diarrhea, rectal bleeding, and general misery. The flare-up lasted for about four months. I had just been given a colonoscopy and prescribed medication to put my colitis back into remission, when I decided to try an alternative, more holistic solution.

Basically, I changed my eating habits (which I fully admit weren't great, even though I was pretty active), and switched to a whole food, organic, mostly plant-based diet.

I decided to adopt the new eating plan immediately. Within three weeks, I lost thirteen pounds and my stomach felt much better. I did end up taking the medication prescribed to me around this point in order to stop the rectal bleeding, but once that was taken care of, I stopped taking it, and continued to improve by simply eating whole, plant-based food.

Both my husband and I agree that eating this way contributed greatly to the huge improvement in my digestive health, as well as the weight loss. We will both continue to eat whole, organic foods and tons of vegetables.

Chapter 6

A Pitch for Plant-Based

"Nothing will benefit human health and increase the chances for survival of life on earth as much as the evolution to a vegetarian diet."[74]

—Albert Einstein

Heads up: this topic is a sensitive one, and this chapter might be a little rough. One of the major reasons it is so difficult to achieve a calm, controlled conversation about plant-based eating with meat eaters, is because the person in the group who doesn't eat animals is inevitably placing unintended blame and guilt upon the omnivorous members of that group. By telling someone that you don't eat meat because it's unethical, for example, implies that those who don't share your view are themselves devoid of ethics. If you were to say that it is because you want to take better care of the environment, or help feed the starving people in the world by taking a stance against the expensive and destructive business of producing and consuming meat, you indirectly blame others for planetary destruction and allowing fellow human beings to go hungry. If you say it's because meat isn't good for you, you are basically inferring that your fellow conversation members are unhealthy people. This is a heated and passionate topic, because there are so many personal biases and experiences that come out to play ball.

That being said, we are totally going to go there.

If you're living with digestive problems, than you should definitely give plant-based eating a go, simply because plants are easier to digest, and proven a healthier alternative to animal meat. The reason I gave up most animal products was for this exact reason. However, since doing so, and researching vegetarianism and all it entails, I have solidified more reasons for myself to remain meat-free. Because I strongly advocate for plant-based eating in this book, my desire is for you to look for even more reasons to go veg. I feel as though the more incentives that are provided for you to adopt the plant-based part of the plan, the better the chance that you might stick with it, and the clearer your mind may be when confronted with skeptical friends and family, or those less educated in the benefits of plant-based nutrition. So, in the hopes of making a well-rounded and convincing argument for adopting a plant-based diet (other than the elimination of chronic stomach pain), I have outlined some major reasons to stop eating meat, and start a lifestyle change that as you will see, will greatly improve your whole life for the better.

Here goes something . . .

Defining "Plant-Based"

So, what exactly does it mean to follow a plant-based diet? Most people think of this act as vegetarianism, and it is usually referred to as the elimination of animal products from one's diet. However, there are different degrees in which a person goes about doing this. There are lacto-vegetarians, who don't eat animal meat (including fish) or eggs, but do consume dairy. (Often because eating these animal products does not directly impact whether an animal lives or dies). There are ovo-vegetarians, who abstain from meat and dairy, but do eat eggs. There are lacto-ovo vegetarians, who do not eat any animal flesh, but do dabble with dairy and eggs from time to time. Pescetarians abstain from all animal meat, except seafood. Last, but certainly not least, a vegan completely abstains from not only animal flesh, eggs, and dairy, but also any other animal by-products, such as gelatine and honey.

"Plant-Based" is a looser term. It means that the basis for your diet is composed of plant foods—foods that literally derive from plants. However, it does not sport the label of "vegetarian" or "vegan," which I personally like. I am not compelled to define my diet by what I eat or don't eat, but I do try and stick with foods that are easily digestible, which means the vast majority of them are whole (not processed) and plant-based. If you feel uncomfortable about being labeled "vegetarian" or "vegan," or labeling yourself as such, then don't. Just think "plant-based." If along your path, you happen to adopt a stricter diet that falls into one of the first two categories, then great. If not, no sweat. Just do the best you can, and you'll know when your diet becomes your perfect fit. You won't hurt anymore!

By removing as much meat and other animal products as you can from your diet, you heavily influence your body to become more regular, work more efficiently, wean off all those added hormones and antibiotics, become less acidic and more alkaline, and generally begin to function the way it was designed. This all equals much better health, beginning with optimal digestion. So, in order to begin healing that stressed-out tummy of yours, consider eliminating one of the biggest factors for digestive (dis)ease: animal products.

Here's the deal with going veggie: like Alicia Silverstone says, "it's a kind life."[75] It's easy on your body, your pocketbook, the animals, and the planet. The following are seven distinct arguments for vegetarianism, each directed at what you might consider the most important aspect of adopting a plant-based diet. These arguments are followed by supplementary topics that will hopefully help round-out this chapter.

For the Biology Skeptic

I think deep down, most of us know that regular consumption of red meat is highly correlated with high cholesterol levels and heart disease.[76] One of the first things any physician does when treating a patient that exhibits the symptoms associated with these diseases is to recommend they cut down on eating red meat. If that physician were to take his own advice one step further, and change that suggestion to include all animal products, then you would have the recommendations of the doctors that I wrote about in the previous chapter. Those doctors have changed their patients' entire lives by doing nothing but providing them with fabulous knowledge regarding exactly what foods they should be ingesting, and why. No medications, no surgeries, no problem! It's all about nutrients, baby.

Human beings were created as herbivores and are not built to properly digest animal proteins. Check out your flat teeth, designed for chewing green stuff. We may have four teeth that are relatively pointy, but that's out of a total of thirty-two teeth. Our teeth are very similar to gorillas' teeth, and they are vegetarians. Carnivores, on the other hand, have exclusively sharp, pointy teeth. (All of them. Go take a look in your cat's mouth.) Humans don't have nearly enough stomach acid to process meat properly. Carnivorous animals have more than enough of the required amount of hydrochloric acid for that very purpose, and also possess very short intestinal tracts that allow them to eat and digest very quickly. Their stomachs are also kept at a lower pH of about 1-2,[77] whereas the human stomach functions optimally at about 2-3.5. Our intestinal tracts are approximately twenty-eight feet long (twenty-three in your small intestine, and five in your large), and it takes us up to seventy-two hours to digest any meat we take in, from mouth to colon.

The result of our long intestinal tracts can equal total horror for those of us with that IBS diagnosis. If your intestines are already sluggish, that means that those once-enticing chicken wings can be trapped in there for a very long time before we evacuate them. This is also why we all feel gross and exhausted following a trip to a steakhouse, not to mention being bunged up for days afterward. Anyone out there frequent unzipperers? (You may as well get used to a few made-up words here and there . . . I'm known for those.) You don't have to be! I used to literally yank off my skinny jeans the very second I got home from dinner anywhere, and throw on my yoga pants. Those days, thank goodness, are a thing of the past for me. (Yoga, however, is not!) We may have evolved to be able to process small amounts of animal meat, but a quick evaluation of our anatomy suggests that it was not the original plan.

When you think of processed food, do you conjure up an image of animal products? You should. Meat is extremely processed, from the artificial insemination of the animals, to the feed laced with growth hormones that is supplied to them, to the conventional factory slaughter of them, right down to the way they are packaged and appear on the grocery stores' shelves. In fact, meat might be the *most* processed food available. The process from conception to grocery store shelves is all very unnatural and unhealthy. I urge disbelievers to do a little research and decide just how much this process contributes to their already existing or inevitably impending digestive unease.

"Unless organically and naturally raised, meat and dairy products contain numerous hormones, antibiotics and toxic chemicals."[78]

—Laura J. Knoff, *The Whole-Food Guide to Overcoming Irritable Bowel Syndrome*

For the Dairy Fiend

Dairy is not much better. When a baby is born, their bodies are designed to digest their mother's milk easily. When they are weaned, on average at about twelve months old, their bodies quit making it possible to digest milk. Milk is something that is specifically designed for babies who cannot consume anything else for months, due to underdeveloped digestive systems, and lack of teeth. We don't bottle human breast milk and still drink it into our thirties, right? (Unless you're my brother-in-law, who thought it would be funny to take a swig from my daughter's baby bottle before being informed that the contents was not formula.) Even cows wean . . . the baby calf stops nursing from her mother around age two. After that, no more milk. Nada. She's like, "Here, eat some grass . . . "

Ever wonder why so many people are lactose intolerant? It's because our bodies are not designed to consume lactose, the sugar in dairy, or casein, the protein. It makes us gassy, constipated, irritable, and full of mucous. This is a train wreck for people with irritable bowels of any form. Eliminating dairy from your diet could be your life saver, especially if you live in a country like the United States, which permits antibiotics and growth hormones to be directly injected into conventionally farmed cattle, therefore creating heavily hormone-laced products, and very unnatural, miserable animals. I'm not letting Canada off the hook here. While it's true that Canadian laws are stricter when it comes to these practices, the country's laws make it legal to add both antibiotics and hormones to the cows' feed, unless the products will be certified as organic.

Not only does your body feel funky due to the lactose intolerance, it is becoming antibiotic resistant, one glass of milk at a time. It's also making our hormones go crazy. In fact, Dr. T. Colin Campbell writes "we should not have our children consume diets high in animal based foods."[79] If that's not enough, there are also genetically modified organisms to worry about now. Sheesh!

If you decide that you can't live without milk, try and purchase it organic from grass-fed cows. If you live in the United States, you may be purchasing genetically-engineered hormone milk, or milk that has been labelled with rBGH. Both the United Kingdom and Canada have refused to sell this milk, but the United States' FDA has approved the sale of this engineered milk since 1994, so the U.S.

stocks their grocery stores' shelves both willingly and readily, even though we probably won't fully know or understand the implication of ingesting so many growth hormones until much, much later.

"Based on conclusions on the adverse veterinary effects of rBGH, particularly an increased incidence of mastitis, lameness and reproductive problems, Health Canada reluctantly broke ranks with the U.S. in January 1999, and issued a formal 'notice of non-compliance,' disapproving future sales of rBGH."[80]
—Cancer Prevention Coalition

Even if you live in a country that makes the sale of this hormone-laced milk illegal, the bottom line is that all milk contains lactose, and none of it can be digested properly. So as if there weren't enough arguments that could be made for the avoidance of dairy, let the lactose one sink in for you. If you have a digestive problem, it might very well be your body screaming for the cessation of all those milk products. I know mine did.

For those of you concerned that eliminating dairy will affect your calcium consumption, you can rest assured. You can easily absorb calcium through whole, unprocessed foods like organic broccoli and raw almonds. In fact, numerous studies conclude that women with the lowest risks of osteoporosis and breast cancer reside in Asia. You know, where they don't drink dairy. To be exact, Chinese breast cancer rates are only about "one fifth of those of western women."[81] In North America, where we drink the most milk in the world, we have one of the highest rates of both osteoporosis[82] and breast cancer.[83]

I'll explain the osteoporosis bit. Osteoporosis is a term used to describe low bone density. The lower your bone density, the greater the risk of bone fractures. Calcium helps create and build bone density, hence the association with milk and good bones. Although calcium is indeed present in cow's milk, milk also is an animal food, and therefore creates an acidic reaction within the human body.

When this reaction occurs, your body pulls its resources together to combat the high levels of acidity, and tackles the acidity with calcium. Where does your body go to for calcium? Your bones. So, as you drink milk, and create an inevitably acidic environment, your bones are forced to leech calcium into your body, rendering your bones calcium-deficient. It does the exact opposite of what we have all learned growing up. Milk is *not* good for you, or your bones.[84]

I totally give props to almond, hemp, soy, and brown rice milk. Try substituting your cow milk for one of these on your cereal, in baking, in smoothies, or just drink them straight-up. They are honestly good for you, definitely can't hurt you, and taste delicious. Try and buy organic when you can, especially soy.

Avoiding dairy products will help so much. The solution to managing IBS-C and diverticulitis (as well as many other digestive diseases for that matter), is to keep a clean colon. Not clogging it with mucousy dairy will work wonders for you. You'll be a new person. If this seems extreme to you, try cutting out one food at a time, but you will probably decide for yourself that you'll want to eliminate them all eventually. You will feel *that* good. It took me almost two years to cut out most of this stuff, and I'm still a work in progress. I still indulge in a little cheese sometimes, but I'm always reminded pretty quickly (like, within two hours), why I shouldn't eat it. It's crazy how well you get to know your body, once you get rid of all the crap. (Pun intended.)

I like to akin the feeling you have with being in touch with your body after giving up meat, as the same feeling you have when you're pregnant. Ladies, I know you know what I mean. Remember how in tune you felt with yourself? Even after you had your baby, you noticed things you never noticed before. (You know, you think you feel your baby kicking, but then realize you have no baby in there anymore, so it must be gas?!) That's what it's like when you give up animal products. Nothing's there to impede the awareness that you naturally have for yourself anymore. You feel everything. It's awesome! It creates a soul to body connection that you'll realize you've been missing without even knowing it.

For the Sick and Tired (of undoubtedly being both sick and tired)

" . . . people who ate the most animal-based foods got the most chronic disease . . . people who ate the most plant-based foods were the healthiest, and tended to avoid chronic disease."
—T. Colin Campbell, PhD and Thomas M. Campbell, MD, *The China Study*

I mentioned before how our bodies were not designed to take in and process animal meat. Some of you might be thinking, "But in caveman days, we ate meat!" This may be true, but we would have eaten way less, and it was definitely not pumped full of weird chemicals. Those lucky animals were not forced to consume grains laden with genetically modified organisms (food, whose DNA has been altered in a laboratory, for the purpose of appearance, extending its shelf life, and its ability to grow in certain conditions), foods no being should ever be fed in the first place. Cavemen *did* hunt, but they also did a lot of gathering and picking (not to mention probably running from things that wanted to eat them), jumping, swimming, and generally moving their tight, muscular caveman bodies all day, every day, in order to survive.

Well, we don't do that anymore (enter pre-packaged, microwavable meals and previously recorded television), and we can no longer digestively process what they did, either. More healthcare professionals than ever before are converging on the conclusion that animal flesh may not be as ideal for human consumption as was once thought. That's big news!

Fresh veggies, fruit, beans, raw nuts, whole grains, and clean, chemical-free water are what our bodies run optimally on. It is a natural, healthy, clean diet that suits our twenty-first century lifestyle perfectly. These nutritious gems are easily digested and eliminated with little or no effort. They easily keep us at our pre-designed, healthy body weight, and they make our skin glow and our hair shiny. They give us energy that lasts all day (say goodbye to that afternoon slump), and they keep our bodies alkaline, not acidic, the latter of which is a breeding ground for disease, and sadly a common one at that. They also provide us with the exact right amount of every vitamin and mineral that we require, and in all the right proportions. No more supplements (except possibly vitamin B12), and no more stress over losing that last ten pounds. A whole food, plant-based diet is the perfect remedy for everything from fatigue, to hormone imbalances, weight loss, and great bowel movements.

Praise the gourd!

If you are currently eating animal products, do you know whether they are factory-farmed, or produced on a smaller scale, organic, family-run farm? If you don't know the answer to this question, then you are eating meat and dairy that are products of a factory-farm. We, by eating this factory-farmed livestock, are plugging our bodies full of antibiotics and hormones that we don't need, and certainly can't process. Do you ever sit back and try and figure out why some antibiotics work on you and not others? Why the teenagers today are so much bigger than the teenagers of forty, or even twenty years ago? Why girls start their periods younger than ever?[85] (It is not uncommon anymore for a nine-year-old girl to begin menstruating.) We have no idea what these toxic substances are doing to us, but we do know that they are neither researched well enough, nor helpful for maintaining good health. Why risk it?

Another issue that falls into this category is the ever-increasing enormous catastrophe of overcrowded hospitals, due in large part to chronic disease and bad immune function. Both of these ailments can be altered for the better by following a healthy, plant-strong diet.

In case you need proof, here is a story that coincidentally happened to be on the front page of my newspaper on the day I was writing this sentence: "Experts Probe Hospital Overcrowding."[86] I'm not sure what needs to be "probed." The answer is fairly obvious. We are sicker than ever before, due to the current disease epidemic in North America, but make no mistake: we, to a large extent, bring this on ourselves.

We are not listening to our bodies screaming for more nourishment and less filler. That's not to say that we don't have some major assistance in making bad food choices. With all the advertising mediums available to us, we absorb a lot of straight-up bullshit from food companies that have a huge stake in you purchasing their substandard product. But how would you even really know it's substandard? The packages have pictures of happy animals, living on green farms, being cared for by smiling farmers. Or perhaps it's a sugary cereal product, with artificial flavors and colors, which now advertises "whole grains" even though there is absolutely nothing "whole" about it. What about water that is advertised as containing added vitamins? With almost as much added sugar as a soda, and just as many artificial colors and flavors, what's healthy about this product that is marketed as such? It's easy to lose sight of what's real and what's a total, obvious, lack of responsibility on the part of these food companies who are purposely deceitful in order to make a little moolah.

Here's a quote from the above mentioned article: "A multi-pronged strategy was rolled out fall 2011 to clear hospital beds faster; reduce lengths of stay, and discharge more elderly patients to home care rather than residential care home."[87] Translation: get sick people in and out as quickly as possible, and let the elderly go home to fend for themselves so that we can save money. Sounds extreme, but is it? This way of thinking doesn't make sense. Should we not be coming up with solutions to make people healthier from the ground up, instead of trying to cut costs while dealing with the aftermath of bad decisions regarding healthcare? Wouldn't a pre-emptive solution be a better way of solving this ever-increasing issue of poor health—the results of the popular western diet that is high in chemicals, and low in nutrients?

The western diet is like the popular girl in high school with whom everyone wants to be friends. The thing is she doesn't care about you. She doesn't even like you. In fact, she's a straight-up backstabbing bitch who'd steal your boyfriend before you even knew what happened!

Like the vast majority of today's food, animals are grown and processed in ways that encourage incredible, undeniable increasing levels of chemicals, hormones, and deadly pathogens. While most processed foods are stripped of nutrients, enhanced with artificial colors, flavors, and stabilizers, and completely over-packaged in warehouses hundreds and even thousands of miles away from where you will actually consume it, animal meat goes one step further. Approximately fifty percent of this meat (yes, I said *half*), is contaminated with harmful bacteria like *E. coli, Listeria, Campylobacter,* and *Salmonella* that can be (and has been) lethal if ingested.[88] Knowing this, you can begin to get an idea of what your digestive system is being subjected to when forced to try and process this type of food.

We are not doing ourselves any favors here. The time has come to take charge of our health. I want to be absolutely certain that I am doing everything I can to make sure my tummy has an easy time on the digestion front, so that if I do become sick, because of reasons beyond my control, I can be assured a hospital bed, in a hospital room, and not in a nearby fast-food restaurant.[89]

For the Frugal

"The greatest wealth is health."[90]

—Virgil

You might be thinking that eating healthily is expensive business, but I argue that you have to be informed of the whole picture. First of all, meat is expensive. Even when it's cheap it's expensive. This is because the price we pay at the grocery store or fast food outlet does not accurately reflect the actual cost of meat.

Meat is heavily subsidized by the government, and we pay only a tiny portion of what it costs to produce an eight ounce steak. If you take into account the cost of grain production to feed just one cow, the amount of water it takes to grow that grain and hydrate that cow, the amount of antibiotics that are pumped into the cow to keep it alive in even ideal situations, the cost of slaughter, and the cost of bringing that meat to your friendly neighbourhood grocery store, the total cost is immense. In fact, if you factor in the amount of money we spend on healthcare for heart disease, high cholesterol, and high blood pressure that's in large part caused by eating all of that beef, the total cost of consuming a single steak is completely insane.

America's healthcare system (and Canada's too, for that matter) is in jeopardy. Although they are both very different systems of health, the United States and Canada have a similar issue that is directly related to the root cause of the core struggle: terrible nutrition. Food that is void of nutrients is the norm in these two countries, and it is this issue that is the main cause for diseases of affluence. Are you interested to know the single most important contribution you can make to help our healthcare system flourish? You guessed it! Eat whole, and plant-based. Disease prevention equals money saved, my friends.

"Vegetarians have the best diet. They have the lowest rates of coronary disease of any group in the country. . . . Some people scoff at vegetarians, but they have a fraction of our heart attack rate and

67

they have only 40 percent of our cancer rate. They outlive other men by about six years now."[91]

—Dr. William Castelli, M.D.

Contrary to meat, vegetables are *inexpensive*. So are grains, seeds, nuts, and beans. Even if you purchase the very best organic, raw foods from the bulk bin (a bag of organic, raw almonds could run about $20), it's still cheaper than buying meat in comparison, because the nuts last a long time. That four-pack of chicken breasts that cost you $20 will only last you a couple of meals, right? If you took the money that you spent on that poultry, and purchased the foods that I'm advocating for now, they would last much longer than a couple of meals. Try a couple of weeks! Those $20 almonds sit in my freezer for about a month. Want to compare the price of a salad at your favorite restaurant to a steak? Didn't think so. Here are ten great tips to help save money when eating a whole, plant-strong diet:

1. Buy bulk. All of your raw seeds, nuts, dried fruit, whole grains, and dried beans can be purchased from the bulk bin. These foods make up a very large portion of a plant-based diet, so all of this in bulk equals tons of savings. Store the nuts and seeds in your freezer to keep them fresh for longer. They taste better this way!

2. Buy in season. The vast majority of your produce should be in season, because it's way cheaper, not to mention healthier. It can be grown locally, so less transport time equals more retained nutrients.

3. Although organic is considerably better for you, there are some fruits and vegetables that you can get away with, without having the organic label. Namely, anything that has a peel that is removed before you eat it. Although there are no guarantees that the seed itself was not genetically modified, you can feel good about knowing that pesticide

sprays did not affect the fruit inside the peel as much as it would have if the peel wasn't present. (The spray still gets in there sometimes, though.) Avocados, bananas, oranges, lemons, limes, melons, coconuts, and mangoes are a few examples of what I'm talking about. Although being sprayed, the peel protects the fruit to a large extent. You can also refer to the "Dirty Dozen" list in chapter ten.

4. Grow your own vegetable garden. For the price of a few packets of organic seeds (Martha Stewart's are around $2.99 per packet), and an hour's worth of weekly maintenance, you can grow your own organic vegetables for months throughout the year. You can spend fifty dollars in seeds, and hope to have loads of free, organic produce, such as beans, beets, carrots, cucumbers, fennel, lettuce, onions, peas, tomatoes, and radishes and from June until October. That's about ten dollars a month for organic veggies! Then, you can plant again in October, and have different veggies available to you, such as arugula, beets, broccoli, brussel sprouts, cabbage, carrots, cauliflower, chard, garlic, kale, onions, potatoes, and squash from January to April.

5. Only purchase what you can eat. In other words, don't let spoilable food go to waste—that would literally be composting or garborating your well-earned cash. Instead, try to shop twice a week, and get inventive so that nothing goes to waste. If something is going to spoil, then freeze it, bake with it, or juice it before it can. As a last resort, throw it in your compost and let it live on in a worm sanctuary.

6. Hit up the farmer's markets. You can get loads of fresh, local, in-season produce for much less than grocery store prices. From May until October, farmer's markets are definitely the way to go. If your community sports a winter farmer's market, then take advantage of it—you're lucky.

7. U-pick your fruit. In the summertime, visit local u-pick farms. You can get all sorts of berries, apples, pears, apricots,

peaches, and plums from farms that let you pick your own fruit, and then pay for it at a very discounted price to account for your labour. Also, it's fun, and a great family outing. Freeze a bunch of it if the quantities you are taking home are too much for your family to eat before it spoils. You can use the frozen fruit for baking, smoothies, or to make homemade popsicles.

8. Avoid highly processed vegetarian fare and meat alternatives, if you can. They are not as good for you, and they cost more. Items like canned beans are a more inexpensive way to go if you're looking for something fast and nutritious. You can use them to make veggie chili, veggie tacos, burritos, soups, and throw them on salads. They are a cheap, yet invaluable source of fiber and protein- a must for a vegetarian diet. Just make sure that you buy cans of food that are labelled "BPA Free." (BPA is an acronym for Bisphenol A, which is chemical compound found in hard plastics and the coatings of aluminum food cans. It has officially been deemed a toxic substance in Canada since 2010,[92] and has been removed from items such as baby bottles and toddler sippy cups in the United States since 2012.[93])

9. Sprout your own sprouts, and grow your own herbs. I used to buy sprouts and herbs every week when I picked up my produce...not anymore! When I figured out how ridiculously easy it is to do these things myself, I never looked back. You can have your own sprouts in three to seven days, and fresh herbs are totally different than the ones you purchase. Plus, they make your kitchen smell amazing!

10. Shop sales. Keep a constant eye out for sales on things like nut butters, almond or brown rice milk, and any supplements you are taking (like digestive enzymes or probiotics), organic teas, fair-trade dark chocolate, or any yummy snack that you have become fond of. Try and buy your pantry staples this way, and you'll save a lot of money.

"Every time you spend money, you're casting a vote for the kind of world you want."[94]

—Anna Lappé, author, educator, sustainable food advocate

If you are still feeling as if a healthier diet could cost you more, ask yourself how much you would pay to rid yourself of digestive unease. Tell yourself that you are investing in your health, and better quality of life, and that you're worth every penny. If ever there was a time to eat a whole food, plant-based diet, it's now. Spend your time and money on being the healthiest, hottest you that you can be, not on substandard food products that make you sick.

For the Humanitarian

"About 2,000 pounds of grains must be supplied to livestock in order to produce enough meat and other livestock products to support a person for a year, whereas 400 pounds of grain eaten directly will support a person for a year. Thus, a given quantity of grain eaten directly will feed 5 times as many people as it will if it is eaten indirectly by humans in the form of livestock products."[95]

—M.E. Ensminger, PhD

It's a little mind-boggling to read the above statistics and realize that by choosing to eat certain foods, you are affecting the ability of others to either eat more or less; people you have never met and probably never will. By avoiding factory-farmed meat, you are reducing the insane amount of grain (particularly corn and soy), and clean water used every year to feed and water livestock, and hopefully place it back into the mouths of hungry people everywhere. I find this reason to forgo animal products such an amazing incentive.

This subject also has to do with the improvement of digestive health that we would all be taking part in by giving up substandard meat, produced by substandard farms. By taking a stand against factory-farmed meat production by avoiding these animal products, you are not only doing your own body a favor, but you are also silently demonstrating for the bodies of those who need that water the most.

In 2010, there were 925 million people who were hungry on our planet.[96] That number has only gotten bigger, and will continue to grow. People for the Ethical Treatment of Animals (PETA) say this:

"There is more than enough food in the world to feed the entire human population. So why are . . . people still going hungry? Our meat-based diet is largely to blame. We funnel huge amounts of grain, soybeans, and corn through all the animals we use for food instead of feeding starving humans. If we stopped intensively breeding farmed animals and grew crops to feed humans instead, we could easily feed everyone on the planet with healthy and affordable vegetarian foods."[97]

For the Environmentalist

"Vegans, whether they eat local or imported food, can boast that their diets use 90% less energy than the average American's . . . "[98]
—Peter Ladner, *The Urban Food Revolution*

By switching to a plant-based diet, you are inadvertently participating in the single most important thing you can do for our planet. It's pretty amazing, and ridiculously easy.

If you are someone who is diligent about upgrading your compact fluorescents to LCDs, recycling your newspapers, composting your organic food remnants, driving a hybrid vehicle or carpooling, using green cleaning products, collecting rainwater for reuse in the garden, keeping a keen eye on your family's water consumption, and/or donating unused or unwanted food to your local food bank, then listen up: going vegetarian will do way more for the environment than all of those things *combined*.

"Food production, processing, and delivery are the greatest threats to environmental health."[99]

—Brendan Brazier, *The Thrive Diet*

In terms of environmental activism, most people who are even semi-conscious about what is happening to our planet are willing to step up and help, even in small ways. For example, I personally do not know anyone who doesn't recycle their water bottles and newspapers. We all know recycling is a good alternative to just throwing things in the garbage, so we all generally participate in that one aspect of environmentalism. There are millions of people who are making more sustainable choices, and feel as though they should. Some choices cost little (such as the price for recycling bags), and some are larger (like the price tag on a hybrid vehicle).

Going vegetarian can have the largest environmental impact, without costing you a dime.[100] In fact, it saves you, and our healthcare system, a lot of dough. Even eliminating half the meat from your diet can have a hugely positive impact on your health, our environment, and your pocketbook. Start slowly if you need to, eating meat only every other day, and notice the change it makes to your insides and your grocery bill. You won't notice the immediate difference that it has on the environment, save for the decrease in food packaging in your garbage bags, but it's definitely there. Here's PETA's opinion: "A recent United Nations report concluded that a global shift toward a vegan diet is necessary to combat the worst effects of climate change. And the U.N. is not alone in its analysis. Researchers at the University of Chicago concluded that switching from a standard American diet to a vegan diet is more effective in the fight against climate change than switching from a standard American car to a hybrid. And a German study conducted in 2008 concluded that a meat-eater's diet is responsible for more than seven times as much greenhouse-gas emissions as a vegan's diet is. The verdict is in: If you care about the environment, one of the single most effective things that you can do to save it is to adopt a vegan diet."[101]

By adopting a plant-based diet, you will make significant steps in repairing your digestive tract and general health. We have absolutely proven that such a diet is very low in trans-fat, saturated fat, cholesterol, and calories, and incredibly high in essential nutrients, fiber, oxygen, vitamins, minerals, and availability. Plus, it's great for the environment, it's cheaper, it's cleaner, and more. Read on, future veggie lovers, read on . . .

For Those Concerned with Animal Welfare

There are many problems that arise from both the treatment of animals in most factory farms, as well as the conditions of these farms in general, that I feel directly relate to human health, and more specifically, digestive unease. This section is going to make a case for adopting a stricter vegetarian diet, or at the very least for purchasing your food animals from local, family-owned, organic farms by shedding some light on why factory-farmed animals are simply not as good for you, or your gut.

"The *eat with care* ethic didn't become obsolete over time, but died suddenly. It was killed, actually."[102]

—Jonathan Safran Foer, *Eating Animals*

Factory-Farms versus Smaller, Family-Run Farms

I have been living in British Columbia's fertile Fraser Valley since the mid-1990s, but I've only recently become amazed at just how many farms are within a thirty-minute radius of my house. I know that the area is well-known for being an agricultural epicenter, but when I really started to pay attention to all of the farm buildings, I was astounded. It's easy to recognize traditional-looking farms. There are rolling pastures, fences, little barns for the animals to shelter themselves in, and of course, the animals themselves are typically clearly visible.

What I have more recently become aware of is just how many farms don't look like farms. These types of operations are easier to spot, now that I know what I'm looking for. To be specific, they are very long, metal buildings; usually two or three of them in a row. There is no sign of actual animals, and often an offensive smell associated with them because of the severe overcrowding that occurs within.

A viable alternative to purchasing and consuming factory-farmed animal products, is to purchase your meat and eggs (and possibly dairy) from a family-run, organic farm. (Visit www.eatwild.com to find one near you—the website offers locations throughout the United States and Canada.)

Exactly nine minutes from my front door is one such farm. The owners of Sumas Mountain Farms[103] work their own land and care for their own animals, along with the help of their children. The farm is organic, SPCA (Society for the Prevention of Cruelty to Animals) certified, and grass-fed and "finished." In essence, this means that besides the organic health benefit to consumers, and the SPCA approved care that their animals are given, animals from this particular farm are allowed to graze naturally, on organic pasture, for their entire lives. The farm also keeps chickens, turkeys and pigs. Their breeds are heritage, which means that their animals have never had their genes manipulated like 99% of today's farmed animals. The owners even transport their own animals to slaughter, to make sure that they are fed and properly hydrated while they wait, unlike the other conventionally-farmed animals there. They also put down hay for them to provide comfort and familiarity. They do this for the sole purpose of being humane to the animals that they have cared for since birth.

One of the owners confided to me that her husband has always been concerned with animal rights, and was even a near-vegetarian before owning their own farm. Their family eats what they raise, because they know exactly what they're consuming. This is important to them, because they know what a conventional farm is about, how it's run, and how the quality of the meat produced there compares to what their own farm provides. They offer a fabulous model of what modern-day animal farming should consist.

The practice of issuing this type of care to food animals greatly enhances the probability that disease does not show up on your plate, which is one more added bonus for those of us suffering from digestive malfunction. Although I personally don't eat very many animal products anymore (I abstain completely from all land animals and most dairy products), I feel comfortable supporting these farms, and having my family consume products from them. It's a good alternative solution.

The typical factory farm operates a little differently. Cows are numbered, not named. Calves are separated from their mothers almost immediately after birth, and instead of being permitted to nurse naturally, they are fed artificial nutrients in a bottle by a farmhand. Dairy cows live for only a few years as long as they are producing milk, and are often treated for exhaustion and infection after the regular doses of antibiotics used to treat their various infections (such as mastitis) stop working. If they are male, they are chained and caged so that they cannot stand up, resulting in underdeveloped calf and thigh muscles. This is done purposely to encourage softer, more tender cuts of veal, which is what these baby calves end up becoming after being slaughtered following a mere four months of life.

When I was about twenty years old, my then-boyfriend and I decided to drive up north to stay with his folks for a few days. We arrived there around dinner, and it wasn't until the next morning that I really noticed the cows. There were probably about eighty of them, all young, which were kept in two long rows of individual stalls about the size of the calves themselves. I remember feeling uncomfortable at the sight of this, but it was my first experience of the type, and it was before I had ever really given much thought to the treatment of farmed animals, as being directly related to the food served up on our plates.

My boyfriend's siblings went out to feed them that morning, and took me along to see what they did. Each of the calves was fed a formula-type mixture from a bottle, and they explained that they would routinely add antibiotics to this mixture so that the cows did not get sick, "like *that* one." I turned my head to the direction they were pointing and saw one of his siblings, around fifteen years old, driving a small tractor that was pulling a presumably dead calf by a rope tied to its leg. This I remember as being completely horrifying to me. Even if the animal was indeed dead, the way in which this poor animal was being treated was shocking to say the least.

"Downers" is the term used for animals that are decidedly too sick or weak or dead to be of use, and so they are piled up, often still alive, while they wait to be disposed of.

Farm Sanctuary, the largest place of rescue in the United States for farm animals to live out the rest of their lives after being discarded by feed lots, was founded by Gene Baur.[104] Baur is an animal rights activist who happened to stumble upon a pile of downers while visiting the Lancaster stockyard one day in the 80s. He noticed how a sheep that he had presumed dead raised her head to look at him. He was so surprised that the animal was alive that he quickly placed her in the back of his vehicle and took off to a veterinarian. He recalls how that sheep lived for ten years after he saved her.[105]

The point is, downers can often be well enough to get better, but finding that out is just not the factory farms' prerogative. A stockyard would rather write an animal off, even though they're sometimes only dehydrated from transport, than stick around to find out. It's a small glimpse into the way factory farming offers cruel and inhumane treatment to food animals.

Back to my personal story, this was my first experience in which it became so terribly obvious that we disassociate these animals and their often horrendous experiences with the food that we buy, cook, and proceed to eat every day.

"When we eat factory-farmed meat we live, literally, on tortured flesh. Increasingly, that tortured flesh is becoming our own."[106]
—Jonathan Safran Foer, *Eating Animals*

It's not just cattle, either. Baby chicks, at only a couple of days old, routinely get their sensitive beaks sheared off to prevent them from pecking each other from stress and frustration. The greater population is incredibly disease-ridden due to severe overcrowding, and many suffer from fatty liver disease from being fed grains that they were never meant to ingest, let alone digest. The stress of the situation often leads to heart failure, and results in death. Factory-farmed chickens are fatter now in a month and a half than they were previously in three months, thanks to the cocktail of growth hormones that is mixed into their feed. This causes great stress to their organs, and they often cannot stand for longer than a minute at a time, because they are incapable of holding up their own body weight. As a result of this, their legs are often completely deformed, and they are typically in chronic pain. Male layers (the male offspring of egg-laying hens) are all destroyed, because they are not broiler chickens (those fattened up to eat), and they cannot produce eggs, so they can't be layers, either.

Each year, approximately 100 million male chicks are killed because they have no use to the chicken industry.[107]

The high percentage of diseased birds that lay eggs that are consumed by the average consumer is alarming. If you knew that the eggs you were purchasing came from diseased and distressed hens, would you still buy them? Eggs that do not come from hens that are permitted to walk around outdoors and peck at the natural ground cover are not kind to your tummy. They typically originate from diseased birds, and contain genetically modified ingredients, antibiotics, and other stuff that most of us would prefer not be there.

Pigs are no happier. Although being incredibly intelligent and social animals by nature, they live their lives in tiny, metal pens, surrounded by their collective feces. Gestation crates are crates made of metal bars that pregnant sows are typically kept in for the entire length of their three months, three weeks, and three day pregnancies. They are so compact that the sow can barely move, and cannot turn around. The common farmer's defense for a gestation crate is that they feel it lessens the likelihood of the sow trampling her piglets. It's "saving her from herself." This is ridiculous and offensive as a fellow female! If the sow had space, like they do in the wild, they would not get nervous and stressed, and subsequently would not squash their young. The situation that these farmers place the sows in is directly related to the outcome of the sow's new piglets. It's the situation itself that creates inevitable stress.

Manure Lagoons

Here's a fun question for you: where does the animal poop go? This topic has serious implications for human heath, even if you don't live next to a factory farm. Waste removal is an enormous issue for these farms. The amount of waste produced on each factory farm is similar to what is produced in a small city. Where cities have environmentally approved waste removal strategies for their citizens, these crowded, fast-paced operations can't possibly provide as such for their food animals. While better waste-removal practices definitely exist, much of the liquid waste that is produced in both Canadian and American farms is moved to above ground storage units, or uncovered lagoons,[108] and eventually an attempt is made to spread the waste back onto fields to be used as fertilizer. This is especially true with hog farms.

There are problems with this. The first is that there is just way too much waste to deal with. The toxic manure can seep into the ground and contaminate soil, ground water, and the air we breathe. The Natural Resources Defense Council and Clean Water Network have come up with, in their view, a list of major reasons why we should all be concerned, with regards to how factory farms dispose of their waste:[109]

1. "Toxic air emissions are making people sick." Hazardous, organic compounds are being released into the air surrounding factory farms, affecting farmers, residents, neighbours, and the animals themselves. These compounds include, but are not limited to, ammonia, hydrogen sulphide, and methane gas.

2. "Pathogens in manure cause human diseases." Swine lagoons contain crazy levels of viruses and bacteria. These pathogens are polluting drinking water, streams, rivers, and creeks, which also affect aquatic life. The diseases and symptoms that humans can contract from living near one of these lagoons includes kidney failure, severe stomach cramps, nausea, diarrhea, fevers, and even death. I definitely recommend finding out where your water comes from, and if its location is close to a swine lagoon.

3. "Nitrates from animal waste pollute drinking water." Nitrates are highly toxic. They are found in many places, but are always present in swine lagoons. When a lagoon seeps, spills, or leaks (which is not rare), those nitrates make their way to nearby drinking water wells. They have been found to cause such issues as spontaneous abortions, developmental deficiencies, or even death in infants. 34% of North Carolina drinking wells near factory farms were found contaminated with nitrates in 1998.[110]

4. "Widespread Use of Antibiotics at Factory Farms Contributes to Antibiotic-resistance." 24.6 million pounds of antibiotics are used annually to treat factory-farmed animals, sick from overcrowded conditions. We eat that meat. Some antibiotics don't work on us anymore. 'Nuf said.

5. "Health of Factory Farm Neighbors and Workers is Harmed by Lagoons and Sprayfields." Common symptoms that farm

workers and neighbours have experienced because of living in close proximity to hog farms include headaches, sore throats, respiratory problems, burning eyes, depression, nausea, diarrhea, and fatigue. More awesome evidence of emerging health issues.

6. "Environmental Devastation." The number of fish that have been killed due to leakage or spills from manure lagoons is in the billions.

7. "Water Contaminants of Concern." This one needs no explanation. Water is contaminated by its exposure to the high levels of factory farms' fecal output. Gross.

8. "Groundwater Pollution and Depletion." Fairly self-explanatory.

9. "Poor Siting." Many of these structures are located in floodplains, near streams, or sitting over aquifers, and are at high risk of drinking water contamination.

10. "Atmospheric Deposition." The liquidly waste eventually turns to atmospheric ammonia, which is able to travel far distances and cause widespread illness.[111] Fantastic news.

In despite of these reasons, manure lagoons are still routinely used both in the United States and in Canada. The effect that the structures have on human health is well known and documented. Nausea and vomiting, both symptoms of being exposed to the compounds that animal waste produces, is proof that our digestive systems are being affected by this common practice of the attempt to remove factory-farmed waste.

Can't Give up Animal Products?

If you still feel strongly that you just can't give up animal products, then at least pledge to try and make steps to change the quality of the product that you are eating. You can make sure that the meat you choose to purchase has been cultivated humanely, responsibly and sustainably. I'm by no means implying that this is an equal alternative to giving up animal products completely. Your health would be significantly better without them, guaranteed. However, the following is some alternative information for those who are completely put off to the idea of a meat-free existence, and I do understand if you are. If you are going to continue eating animal products, such as meat, eggs, and dairy, here's what you want to look for:

Meat

Many food companies will claim that their products are derived from free range, free run, organic, naturally raised, and/or grass-fed animals. All of these titles are undeniably synonymous with greater health, but don't be fooled. Farms can technically claim that their chickens are "free range" or "free run" when they are not caged, but only have half a square foot of space in which to stand. "Organic" can mean that the corn and soy fed to the animal is, indeed, organic, but overlooks the fact that the animals are still caged, and that they should not eat stuff like corn in the first place. (Most farmed animals should not eat corn. It makes them sick by changing the pH of their stomachs. Corn is not a natural feed for cows, chickens, or pigs.) "Grass-fed" can mean that in one time in a particular cow's life, it ate grass. "Natural" means nothing; it's just a label.

Search for a local farm that is family run, and allows their animals to graze, walk, root, and nest all day long. See it with your own eyes. These animals are typically treated much better than their factory-farmed counterparts, and they are not usually given any growth hormones or antibiotics. They don't need them because they are permitted to live the way they're supposed to, which means they are not in overcrowded conditions, riddled with disease. These animals are handled more carefully, and with pride. You will pay more for this meat, because the farmer is not able to produce the enormous amount of beef produced on a factory farm or feedlot, but it will be much better quality and you will have the satisfaction of knowing that the animal had a good life, and that you are receiving a superior product.

Heads up: the taste and appearance of this meat might be very different from what you have been accustomed to. The taste is (apparently) more wild, dense, and lean, and the appearance is different because it's less processed. For example, pork ribs will not be as polished looking as the ones you can find at your local grocery store, and that could be a little bit shocking. Beef will be leaner because cows graze on grass. Pork will be fattier and more pink in color because pork is naturally higher in fat, and factory farms breed pigs to be lean and their meat to be pale.

Eggs

Like meat, eggs can have a lot of claims associated with them. If you are going to eat eggs, the best solution is to find a local family farm who sells them. The eggs should be from hens that are not caged, and free to roam and peck as they please. You should be able to visibly see them doing so. Again, these hens will not have the need for antibiotics, and their feed is straight from the earth, so no growth hormones or genetically modified ingredients are involved. These eggs are generally not much pricier than what you could buy at the grocery store. If you initially feel that this sounds like a lot of work, please bear in mind that once you have a great contact, you will know where to go from then on. Also, knowing where these products come from, how they are processed, how the animals were treated, and what's in them (or, more importantly, what's *not* in them), will give you immense satisfaction.

Again, I still hold the opinion that consuming zero animal products is best for those in the throes of digestive unease, but the second best option would be this one. As for taste, they taste much better than the supermarket variety, hands down. They are also typically varied in size, shape, and color, because they have not been bred to produce eggs of specific, uniform size. It's also nice to know that the hens themselves are not all deformed and featherless or kept in overcrowded battery cages. These hens have a pretty sweet life in comparison.

Ah, the life of a happy pecker . . .

Dairy

Dairy is difficult. If you think about how milk gets from the cow to our refrigerators, it's tough to make any sort of case for milk, unless you are milking your own cow. (Which is still weird.) Conventional cows' milk is full of antibiotics and hormones, but even worse is the suffering that factory-farmed dairy cows are routinely subjected to. The whole process of industrialized milking is kind of gross.

If you're going to consume dairy while considering the adoption of more humane practices when it comes to food animals, and still working towards the goal of healing your digestive issues, you need to find a farmer who allows her cows to pasture-feed naturally, milks them personally and individually (without the assistance of a large, un-manned machine), and does not keep them perpetually pregnant. They should be given no growth hormones or antibiotics. They should be healthy and happy. If you can find such a farm in your area that offers dairy being derived in this manner, then that's your best bet.

Some people are really into raw (unpasteurized) milk. The major benefit one receives from drinking raw milk instead of pasteurized milk, is that raw milk still holds all of its original nutrients. When milk is pasteurized, most of the original nutrients are killed along with the bacteria that pasteurization is designed to kill. Then, those nutrients are added back into the milk in the form of "added nutrients," or fortification. It's a lose-lose situation in my opinion. Because I truly believe that milk is nowhere near the perfect food for humans, I have a hard time making a case for pasteurized versus raw milk. Pasteurized, technically, does not carry the harmful bacteria that raw milk can, but raw milk is technically less processed and therefore more nutritious than its counterpart.

There's really no good solution on the dairy front. Please remember that cow's milk is for cows, and our bodies cannot handle it well, even if the condition in which the milk is produced is optimal for all parties concerned. I recommend you skip this whole cow milk thing, and go buy yourself some organic, unsweetened almond milk. Yum!

Sad Stats and Freaky Facts: For Those Who Need Proof

"I don't understand why asking people to eat a well-balanced vegetarian diet is considered drastic, while it is medically conservative to cut people open and put them on cholesterol-lowering drugs for the rest of their lives."[112]

—Dean Ornish, MD, Preventative Medical Research Institute

The following information is a compilation of statistics that I have found really makes me question our nation's food choices and ideas about proper health. Many of these stats or facts may seem unreal, yet all are true.

Concerning Our Health

1. "In 1952, just 11% of American corn was treated with pesticides and herbicides; today the statistic is over 95%."[113]
2. "Americans spent almost $300 billion dollars at supermarkets in the past year, with the number one item being carbonated beverages, which clocked in at about $12 billion."[114]
3. "Number of U.S. medical schools: 125. Number requiring a course in nutrition: Thirty."[115]
4. "The number of underfed and malnourished people in the world? 1.2 billion. The number of overfed and malnourished people in the world? 1.2 billion."[116]
5. "More people die because of the way they eat than by tobacco use, accidents or any other lifestyle or environmental factor."[117]

6. "Americans choose to eat less than 0.25% of the known edible food on the planet."[118]

7. "On average, Americans eat the equivalent of 21,000 entire animals in a lifetime."[119] If you take into account the incredibly large percentage of diseased animals that make it through processing, that's an obscene amount of diseased meat that we've all purchased and eaten.

8. (Approximately) "95% of chickens become infected with *E. coli* . . . and between 39–75% of chickens in retail stores are still infected."[120]

9. Historically speaking, we are entering into the first generation of children who may not live as long as, or longer than, their parents. This is due to the sheer prevalence of "western diseases" that are completely preventable by dietary alteration.

The following five statistics are from *Forks Over Knives*; edited by Gene Stone:

1. "Obesity rates for North American children have doubled in the last thirty years."

2. "In the last decade alone, the incidence of diabetes has grown 90%."

3. "70% of deaths in the United States stem from chronic diseases."

4. "Every day, 1500 people die from cancer."

5. "Every minute, somebody in the United States dies from heart disease."[121]

Concerning Animals

1. Egg-laying hens get less space in which to live their "lives" than what constitutes an 8 1/2 x 11 piece of foolscap paper.[122]

2. 99% of meat we eat comes from factory farms.[123] Two generations ago, that statistic was less than 1%.

3. "Number of animals killed for meat per hour in the United States: 660,000."[124]

4. About 95% of America's eggs are produced by chickens living in battery cages.[125]

5. "Each year, hundreds of thousands of pigs arrive at slaughterhouses dead, dying, or diseased."[126]

6. Globally, roughly 70 billion land animals are now factory farmed every year.[127]

7. "Chickens once had a life expectancy of fifteen to twenty years, but the modern broiler is typically killed at around six weeks. Their daily growth rate has increased roughly 400%."[128]

8. Dairy cows only live for about five years before being considered "spent." Calves that will become veal will live for four months. If left alone, allowed to graze naturally in the open air, cows live for upwards of twenty-five years.

9. Most of us are all effectively eating genetically mutated poultry, even when it's free range and "natural." Factory farmed poultry can't even reproduce anymore without scientific intervention.[129]

10. Most cases of the "twenty-four-hour flu" are actually caused by a food-borne pathogen, not influenza.[130]

Concerning the Environment

1. "Omnivores contribute seven times more greenhouse gas emissions than vegans do."[131]

2. "Modern industrial fishing lines can be as long as seventy-five miles—the same distance from sea level to space."[132]

3. "Animal agriculture makes a 40% greater contribution to global warming than all transportation in the world combined; it is the number one cause of climate change."[133]

4. "Years the world's known oil reserves would last if every human ate a meat-centered diet: thirteen. Years they would last if human beings no longer ate meat: 260."[134]

5. "A single dairy cow produces approximately 120 pounds of wet manure a day."[135]

6. "Five tonnes of animal waste is produced for every person in the United States."[136]

7. "On average 16,000 litres of water are required to produce one kilogram of beef."[137]

8. "More than 260 million acres of U.S. forest have been cleared to grow grain for livestock."[138]

9. "Raising chickens, turkeys, pigs and other animals for food causes more greenhouse gas emissions than all the cars, trucks and other forms of transportation combined."[139]

10. "Livestock are one of the most significant contributors to today's most serious environmental problems. Urgent action is required to remedy the situation."[140]

As you can see, there are many ways in which the business of meat production is harmful. While I know firsthand that it might be hard to imagine your life without meat being a major part of your meals, there are so many amazing and compelling reasons to ditch it for good, or to at least find somewhere to purchase better quality fare. Digestive health is definitely affected by our average consumption of factory-farmed animal products, but so are many other things. If you can't give up meat for yourself, maybe you can reduce it as a way of helping out on some of the other causes associated with meat and its production.

Question: What makes the topic of eliminating animal meat and dairy such an emotional and passionate subject for people? Is it a health reason? Is it a question of tradition? Is it a misleading connotation? What does giving up meat and dairy mean to you?

Chapter 7

Filthy Food

Well, this is a super fun topic. However, if you have ever had to endure the symptoms associated with food poisoning, I can guarantee you that it's no laughing matter. An incredibly large portion of food-borne disease is traced back to meat. Remember these?

- 1993: *E. coli* outbreak in Jack-in-the-Box in the Seattle area is responsible for the deaths of four children.[141]
- 1997: *E. coli* outbreak in Colorado involving beef from Hudson Foods.[142]
- 1998: *Listeria* outbreak in Michigan involving Sara Lee products results in twenty-onepeople dead.[143]
- 2008: *Listeria* in lunch meat from Maple Leaf Foods in Toronto kills twenty-three people.[144] Or more recently (and more locally for myself):
- 2012: *E. coli* outbreak in Alberta-based meat packing company forces massive XL Foods recall.[145]

Animal meat itself is not entirely to blame. Mostly it's the animals' living conditions in which they are kept, and the result of careless processing that encourage deadly bacteria, such as *E. coli*, *Salmonella*, *Campylobacter* and *Listeria* to become exposed to meat intended for human consumption. Countries that care for their animals more humanely by permitting them to grass-feed, allowing the implementation of natural grazing habits, and then practicing careful and skillful "kills," have a way lower rate of food-borne disease than countries like the United States and Canada, whose factory-farmed quick and careless form of meat processing is, to put it mildly, very dirty. Animal flesh intended for human consumption becomes contaminated when, during processing, the gut of the animal is accidentally or carelessly sliced, allowing for the bacteria that lives in the animals' intestines to become exposed to other parts of the carcass, or the assembly line on which it's being processed.[146] This happens all the time.

Sometimes it's not the animals' living conditions, or the way in which they are terminated: it's the feed. Unlike humans, cows possess four separate digestive compartments within one stomach. The second compartment is called a rumen, and it's that compartment that I find the most interesting. Its purpose is to ferment grasses in order to digest them better, and more readily absorb the nutrients associated with feeding from the earth. The rumen contains way less acid than our stomachs do, and when *E. coli* passes from the cow to their meat, and in turn to humans who consume that meat, it is usually killed off in our highly acidic digestive tracts.

Well, this is not necessarily the case anymore. For the past few decades, cows being fattened up on feed lots have been routinely fed corn, which has created a huge, unforeseen problem. The corn changes the pH of the rumen, making it more acidic, and *E. coli* is learning to adapt to this acidity. When the pathogen is consumed by humans, it is not being killed off in our stomachs as effectively. As a result of this fairly new situation, we are getting sick.

Remember that particularly terrifying epidemic of Mad Cow Disease that originated in the U.K. in 1986, leaving many people dead after experiencing psychosis from tainted beef products?[147] That horrific situation was essentially caused by cattle being fed feed that contained beef by-products, or bone-meal. Unassuming consumers ate the meat from the infected cows, and now we have a human form of the disease called Creutzfeldt-Jakob disease. The FDA made the practice of feeding cattle beef by-products illegal in 1997.[148] This means that before that year, cows, which are vegetarian animals, were eating their own species, and then we ate that product.

How gross is that?

This scary disease can be passed from infected cows to humans through eating any cow products, including dairy. Symptoms include the breakdown of brain tissue and function, which result in the appearance of severe dementia. What's even more frightening? It can develop over a period of forty years in humans.[149] This leaves me, as well as many others, thinking that maybe there is something more to all of these current forms of dementia being experienced by our grandparents, parents, or partners.

Brain function aside, if you're trying to figure out what food-borne disease has to do with your inflammatory bowel disease, I'll tell you. In *The Food Revolution*, John Robbins writes that "we have learned that many cases of Crohn's disease may be caused by a micro-organism known as MAP (Mycobacterium avium subspecies paratuberculosis) present in cow's milk and not killed by pasteurization."[150] If pathogens are finding their way from the food we eat, to inside our digestive tracts, then it makes perfect sense that a digestive disorder would develop. It is well documented that many cases of IBS begin with a stomach flu or digestive illness of some sort. Maybe it's not a diagnosis of exclusion after all. Maybe it's a simple case of nasty food invaders gone wild! (No, that's not a video game . . .)

Some pathogens have been found in fruits and vegetables too, often by being grown using fecal-contaminated water or by contamination during processing and packaging. However, they are found much more often in animal products. In fact, many meat, egg and dairy distributors blame "food poisoning" on the handling of the food by whoever cooks or prepares it. While it's true that there are proper ways of handing raw animal products, those products need to be infected in the first place. If you knew that the chicken you were purchasing was infected by *Salmonella,* would you still buy it? I'm guessing not. Yet everyday, a great percentage of meat taken home from the grocery store by unsuspecting consumers is infected. Here are some common symptoms of food poisoning:

- Abdominal cramps
- Diarrhea
- Vomiting
- Fever and/or shallow breathing
- Confusion and/or blurred vision
- General shock

By reducing or eliminating your consumption of animal products, you will greatly reduce your risk of ever being exposed to one or more of these dangerous bacteria.

Food Irradiation

Food irradiation was something I had never heard of until I started writing this book. The general public has no idea what this is. This is another example of how, like genetically modified organisms, important decisions are being made for us that concern our food, but there is no real public knowledge regarding the safety of its implementation on our health. At least food that has been irradiated is required to display a symbol (called a "radura") to indicate that it has been as such. Even though there is a symbol for irradiation, not many people know what it means or why it's there. This is the symbol indicating that a particular food has been irradiated: ☻

Essentially, food irradiation is the treatment of some foods with x-rays, electron beams, or gamma rays, as a means of cold pasteurization. The purpose of this procedure is to destroy active bacteria in order to control food-borne disease. Food irradiation has been approved for fruits, vegetables, poultry, red meats, and spices in the United States.[151] In Canada? Wheat, onions, potatoes, flour, spices, and seasonings are all permitted to be irradiated.[152] If a food has been through this procedure, it is obligated to display the international symbol for irradiation, along with a statement saying that it has been irradiated. This, at least, makes it much easier to assess which foods you are eating fall into this category, *if* you know what to look for.

Although both the U.S. Food and Drug Administration[153] and the Canadian Food Inspection Agency have given irradiation the green light in terms of safety,[154] there are many out there who question this practice, including myself. Essentially, your food is being exposed to unnecessary radiation. That's equivalent to your doctor recommending that his or her patients undergo chemotherapy every now and again just in case they have cancer. We all know that radiation of any kind is not that great for you, hence the lead garments they put over your reproductive organs, and thyroid shields that are regularly used during routine dental x-rays. I don't want my food to be irradiated, and I certainly feel that people should be aware that this is becoming standard practice for some foods. If manufacturers are irradiating food to prevent bacterial infections that may cause food poisoning, then you should be aware that food is not sterilized by this practice, nor is it not exposed to bacteria after the irradiation occurs. In other words, even though your food could have been fried for you, it can still harbour harmful bacteria that it picked up afterwards during packaging, storing, handling, etc. The whole practice sounds dangerous, and completely unnecessary.

When making an effort to rid your diet of anything that could be potentially causing you digestive distress, or even anything that just doesn't fall into the category of conscious, clean eating, food that has been irradiated should definitely, in my opinion, be on your radar.

Genetically Modified Organisms

Arran Stephens, author of *The Compassionate Diet*, calls the introduction of GMOs "playing God with our food supply."[155] GMO is an acronym for "genetically modified organism" Unfortunately, you are definitely eating these altered foods. The most common foods that have been genetically modified to date are corn, soy, canola, and cottonseed. When I say "common," I mean that in Canada and the United States, over 90% of these crops are genetically modified.[156] That's insane, considering there has never been any research indicating any level of safety in regards to what these foods might mean to their consumers in terms of long-term health.[157] Other foods that are often modified are papaya, zucchini, alfalfa (hay, not sprouts), and sugar beets.[158]

"Currently, there is no way to monitor the long-term effects of GM food consumption on the population."[159]

—Ontario Public Health Association

The way that genetic modification is connected to gastrointestinal issues is astonishing. Although scientists cannot be certain that GMOs are a major cause of diseases such as IBD, IBS, colon cancer, and other chronic gastrointestinal disorders, it hasn't been disproven, either. If you hear the case for the strong connection, I'm sure it will make you think twice about consuming these products.

One company that has been largely responsible for the genetic modification of our food is Monsanto Corporation. Monsanto has developed such chemicals as Agent Orange and DDT, both highly toxic to humans.[160] They also manufactured the Bovine Growth Hormone (rBGH, the chemical that is added to milk in the United States in order to increase milk production in dairy cows) that was discussed in chapter six. However, they are most widely and recently known for their product called Roundup, and their brilliant subsequent product, Roundup Ready seeds.

Roundup is an herbicide that farmers use to spray their crops with, in order to kill weeds. The active ingredient in Roundup is glyphosate. Glyphosate works by making unwanted weeds diseased.[161] Because most farmers who use Roundup also use Roundup Ready seeds (which are designed to withstand the effects of Roundup), the crops are blanket-sprayed with the herbicide and the farmer does not have to worry about his crop feeling the effects. Sounds like a good idea so far . . .

Roundup Ready seeds are crop seeds, such as corn, that incorporate a gene that codes for Bt toxin,[162] which is designed to rupture the gut of insects that attempt to consume the plants, resulting in death. Essentially, these crops contain built-in pesticides, and the two products together are used to increase crop yields by minimizing damage caused by weeds, insects and other small critters.

Here's the problem: if these foods are designed to carry a chemical responsible for causing intestinal damage in insects, then perhaps we are also susceptible to the effects. Enter the enormous influx of gastrointestinal issues that North America has been facing since the mid-1990s[163] . . . the exact time when genetically engineered foods were introduced to the masses. Is this just a coincidence? We are all consuming those modified crops that have been heavily treated with an obvious poison. Also, most factory-farmed cattle are fed genetically modified corn and soy, or corn and soy that have been sprayed with Roundup. We are getting a double whammy of GM food that has been covered in pesticides and herbicides through our consumption of both produce and factory-farmed meat. It's a cycle of chemicals being infused into our crops, animals, and now us.

What are we doing to ourselves?

A note on "leaky gut": although you may have never heard of this term, "leaky gut" refers to the chronic breaking down

> of the intestinal wall, which causes food particles to escape into the abdominal cavity. One theory on what causes this permeability is the constant inflammation that the intestine experiences when consistently being exposed to toxins, parasites, infection, medication,[164] or food that it recognizes as unfamiliar or foreign. (Often the result of either a poor diet or a food allergy.) Genetically modified foods contain unknown side-effects, which might exacerbate allergies and insensitivities in certain individuals. When in doubt, buy organic!

Our bodies were not designed to recognize genetically modified organisms. This creates a panic in our immune system that leads to inflammation. As you read in chapter four, inflammation is the leading cause of chronic disease. Monsanto engineered a way, in just two decades, to synthetically engineer almost all of America's corn and soy supply.[165] Just for big-picture clarification, there is corn and/or soy in almost all processed foods. That means that if you are eating processed food on a regular basis, along with 90% of Canada and the United States' population, you are consistently consuming genetically modified organisms. Again, we have no idea what this means for our health, or that of future generations. In *No Happy Cows*, John Robbins writes "tens of millions of people are unknowingly eating these inadequately researched foods daily. It's a mass experiment, except that there is no control group."[166]

GM foods are scary. If my lunch has anything to do with a scientist holding a test tube, I'm out. Even though Monsanto claims that these products are not harmful, they also made such claims about their other best-sellers, DDT, Agent Orange, and rBGH. (Remember the slogan, "DDT is good for me?!")[167] Is there any coincidence that The United States and Canada have become home to these relatively new western diseases that are now so mainstream?

All Drugged Up

While antibiotics are definitely important, they have their time and place. If you have an infection that absolutely will not go away on its own, or if you have a serious situation in which antibiotics are a must, then that is when they should be used. Unfortunately, they are not only used in those situations, and because of our blatant overuse of them (sigh), we are now in trouble. (I'm sure there are Canadians reading this and thinking of Canada's "Not all bugs need drugs!" campaign.)

Many of us are guilty of making a beeline to our family doctor or walk-in-clinic and demanding antibiotics at the first sign of a sniffle or cough, and too many doctors just hand them right over. It's that easy. The problem with today's ridiculous overuse of antibiotics is serious. More and more bacteria are becoming antibiotic resistant, which means a large variety of these life-saving concoctions are becoming useless. It also means that people are more and more commonly being treated with two or three rounds of antibiotics in order for their infections to be successfully treated.

This, in turn, wreaks major havoc on our intestinal flora. Antibiotics kill all bacteria; good and bad. Our tummies harbor millions of good bacteria, designed to break down food. If all that bacteria is slain through routine use of antibiotics, our guts get thrown off their delicate balance, which is why antibiotics are routinely known to cause things like diarrhea, nausea, and yeast infections.

If you are suffering from a chronic digestive disease, particularly one that can cause routine infections, such as diverticulitis or IBD (colitis or Crohn's disease), then you are no stranger to antibiotics. But this situation creates an awful circle of events . . . having to treat an infection with antibiotics, only to leave your immune system thrashed from it (most of your immune function comes from your gut),[168] which finally leads you to a predisposition to more infection.

To make matters worse, if you are eating meat or consuming dairy, then you are getting a double, triple, or maybe even a quadruple dosage of these antibiotics, depending on where you buy your meat. Factory farming is a breeding ground for disease largely due to overcrowding and fecal contamination. That means that antibiotics are routinely being pumped into cows, chickens, and pigs in every feed, in order to keep them alive to either be productive, or until they get mature enough to slaughter. In fact, farmers routinely treat these animals *before* they get sick, because they know that their animals' chances of contracting disease is extremely high given the conditions in which they are forced to live.

"In the United States, about 3 million pounds of antibiotics are given to humans each year, but a whopping 17.8 million pounds are fed to livestock . . . "[169]

—Jonathan Safran Foer, *Eating Animals*

By adopting a plant-based diet, you will cut down on your own need for antibiotics, because your healthy, high-fiber, light way of eating will ensure a proper digestive process, including regular elimination. You will also cut down your consumption of these overused drugs by not ingesting them through animal products. This will keep that gut flora in check and your digestive system happy and healthy. It's a win-win situation. As of July 2013, I have not had the need for antibiotics since cutting most animal products out of my diet. Not even once.

If you do need to take antibiotics, then make sure that you use them correctly. If you feel better after taking half of it, and stop taking them, then you are inadvertently leaving your body prone to bigger, better bugs because chances are, not all of those bugs were killed off. The army resurges! Take the entire prescription. Also, when you are done, please treat yourself to a twice-daily dose of probiotics for a week, to help build up the good bacteria again. The good stuff is important!

It is becoming more common than not to consume foods that have been irradiated, genetically modified, and laced with loads of antibiotics. By being more diligent about our food purchases, we have the power to avoid consuming such filthy food. These food practices just sound like bad ideas designed to make life easier for those getting rich on feeding our country sub-standard, shady food.

Question: If you knew that your food was irradiated, genetically modified, or pumped full of antibiotics, would you still purchase them?

Highlight: Jeff's Story

As a child, I always had a sensitive stomach. My diet did not include a great variety of fruit, raw vegetables, or healthy fiber choices. As I became a teenager, the situation grew more severe. The scope of my food intake became even smaller as I started to experience extreme stomach pain, often causing me to sit out from sports and miss school. The situation continued to get worse, and I began to seek the advice from doctors and specialists. This culminated with emergency visits to the hospital, and then eventually I was admitted to Vancouver Children's Hospital for surgery. There, I underwent many tests emerging with the official diagnosis of Crohn's disease.

After being released from the hospital, I was placed on a complex series of medications and the situation became less severe with the bouts of discomfort being less intense.

I continued to suffer moderately through my teen years and into early adulthood, and it was not until I was in my late twenties that the effects of a proper diet really began to become obvious.

I continued to notice a change as I eliminated more and more processed foods, with my attention turning to vegetarian and raw choices. Because of this change in both my diet and myattitude towards food in general, I am happy to say that I have been problem and medication free now for many, many years.

Chapter 8

Chemically Speaking . . .

T he definition of food: "material consisting essentially of protein, carbohydrate, and fat used in the body of an organism to sustain growth, repair, and vital processes and to furnish energy; something that nourishes, sustains, or supplies."[170]

Notice how the definition emphasizes the food's ability to sustain growth, repair, furnish energy, and nourish? Now think of fast food, processed food, and all the chemicals tossed into the mix of what's being eaten on a daily basis by the majority of North America.

A significant amount of people are not eating food. They're just eating.

Reductionism is the act of removing targeted nutrients from the whole of one food (extracting calcium from broccoli, for example), and isolating it in order to either market this nutrient by itself in the form of a calcium supplement, or to add it to an existing preparation in order to make it more attractive to the consumer, such as "calcium fortified" orange juice.

The argument for reductionism sounds well intentioned: by adding a nutrient to orange juice that it does not naturally possess, the consumer can take advantage of ingesting that nutrient without having to eat broccoli. Win-win! Except . . .

Recent studies have shown that by removing the nutrient from its original whole food, it does not work as well, if at all.[171] Scientists are beginning to understand that the complexity of that particular nutrient needs the environment of that whole food in order to activate the benefits. For example, perhaps there is an element to the food that helps that nutrient be absorbed when eaten, and without that element, it just won't happen. This could be an "ah-ha moment" for all those who have hailed reductionism as the next best thing since (iron fortified) sliced bread. The result is this: the whole food will always be more nutritious, in every way, than the sum of its parts. For anyone experiencing digestive unease, you already know that we could all definitely benefit from better nutrient absorption.

Crappy Food? If Only!

Let's be real. Processed food, fast food, refined sugar, bleached flour, and not enough healthy drinking water equals major constipation. Realistically, this is the diet of the average North American. We are all, literally, full of shit. You might think you're having good bowel movements, but unless you are regularly moving your bowels without effort, in some significant way, at least once a day, then you are constipated, my friend. Chronic constipation is strongly correlated with IBS, diverticulitis, and colon cancer, and a symptom synonymous with obesity and heart disease. We need to take care of our tummies *and* our tushies! A vegetarian diet that is high in fiber is extremely effective in moving excess stool. All those fresh, raw vegetables and whole grains work their magic and provide some major relief on the bowel-busting front.

Major things to avoid are foods that are not actually . . . food. Anything that comes in a bag or a box is probably not very nutritionally dense. Also, packages that claim to be low in some ingredients and high in nutrients are probably good to avoid. Good food does not need to sell itself. Eggplant does not come with warning labels or stickers that rave about the nutritional value of it.

It doesn't need to, because its eggplant. As in, ingredients: eggplant. That's what it means to be a whole food.

In his very successful book, *In Defense of Food*, Michael Pollan observes that we are currently living in an age of "nutritionism."[172] In other words, our western diet is completely caught up in defining foods by their nutrients, and skipping over the bigger picture—the whole food itself. We all know that eating an apple is better for us than drinking fortified apple juice, and yet we still feel pretty good about ourselves when we pick up that juice, even though its completely devoid of fiber (among other things), which is essential to digestion and only available when you eat the actual apple.

> Juicy info: Juicing your own fruits and veggies is a little different, because even though you still remove the fiber component from the juice, you do get the fresh nutrients if you drink it right away. Raw juice can only retain its original nutrients and enzymes for about thirty minutes, unless you seal it quickly, without air, and still drink it within the day. Juice you buy at the grocery store has nothing living left in it to give. Poor juice!

This totally bizarre way of looking at food has been going on for decades, ever since it was deemed more profitable to market the nutrients of food, instead of the actual whole food. (Back to the apple.) I myself am completely guilty of buying into that concept without even thinking twice about it.

> "Consumed mostly for convenience sake, processed and refined foods have led to a decline in health and to elevated medical costs."[173]
> —Brendan Brazier, *The Thrive Diet*

The problem with nutrients being separated or isolated from the whole food (as Michael Pollan points out), is that we don't even know if they work outside of the original confines of nature. That is, you can mimic a nutrient (such as an antioxidant) and place it in something like a capsule, advertising it as an easy-to-consume, daily dose of antioxidants. However, we don't even know if that nutrient has any health benefits once removed from its original source. Maybe that nutrient is supposed to work in conjunction with other nutrients from the whole food, and once isolated, has no benefit anymore. These are the kind of questions we need to be asking ourselves. An advertisement that comes to mind right now is a current television commercial advertising a leading brand of margarine. The message is that plant sterols are good for you, and they have been added to this margarine, so you should buy and use this product.

Hold up: can't we just eat a plant?

We need to get back to basics, and remember that we all know a lot more about food than we think we do. When we choose a food to consume, we should always ask ourselves whether or not we would feed it to a small child. From a very young age, we were taught that fruits and vegetables were good. We were fed oatmeal as toddlers. Our mothers hydrated us with water in the summertime. Would you let a two-year-old drink a can of soda, or eat a bag of potato chips? I sure hope not! Let's give ourselves the same respect and care that we would give to a two-year-old. Small children aren't the only people that require optimum nourishment; we all do, every single day for our entire lives.

We all scream for ice cream? If your tummy is telling you to skip this popular frozen dessert, then listen to it. Nothing will help your digestion more than a back-to-basics, whole food approach. This is what John Robbins, son and nephew of the founders of Baskin-Robbins did. Robbins decided he wanted nothing to do with the ice cream industry because of many of the same reasons outlined in this book. Instead, he walked away from his family's fortune and wrote *Diet for a New America, The Food*

> *Revolution,* and *No Happy Cows*—three of the most important pieces of today's literature on the topic of food and its correlation with disease. He watched as a diet that included daily servings of ice cream contributed to the death of his uncle (Baskin) in his early fifties, and then again as it played a large role in the many health problems his father (Robbins) experienced, such as high blood pressure and diabetes. John was finally able to convince his father, co-founder of one of the most famous ice cream companies in history, to adopt a plant-based diet in his late seventies.[174]

Umm . . . How Do I Pronounce This?

There are many people who feel uncomfortable about what they are eating, but our western diet is just so mainstream, that real food is portrayed as "health food," and that phrase has a funny connotation attached to it. It's dumbfounding just how so many people can stare at someone eating a beet and endive salad or a bowl of steamed soybeans, and say something like "I'm not eating that . . . that's health food!" To this I would reply, "No, it's food . . . as in, whole vegetables and real, unprocessed ingredients. That bag of chips you're holding, now that's not food. You can't even pronounce what the ingredients are!" Which brings me to my next bit here . . .

First of all, if you don't know what an ingredient is, or can't pronounce it, then I seriously recommend that you don't eat it. Some of these things are known to be composed of carcinogens and other dangerous chemicals that can wreak havoc on your body. Others have not been thoroughly tested, and should make us nervous for what we might find out about them in the future. None of these items need to be included in a healthy diet.

In Your Food

The following list of additives is not conclusive. Processed food is loaded with these ingredients, which help with the preservation, taste, appearance, and overall marketability of crappy, fake food. I dare you to pull a few items out of your pantry and compare this list to the listed ingredients on their boxes. If you are absorbing these chemicals by eating them, then obviously they are going straight to your digestive system, right? They do damage there! We are discovering more and more that these additives are either not tested, "generally recognized as safe"[175] (still so confused about the safety of that title), sort of safe in very small quantities, used to not be labelled as safe but now are, or fully known to be derived of a cancer causing substance. I'm not joking. A recent news story to sweep the United States in 2012 has been the decision to suspend Coke and Pepsi's current recipe of caramel coloring, which has been identified as carcinogenic:

"Coca-Cola Co. and PepsiCo Inc. are changing the way they make the caramel coloring used in their sodas as a result of a California law that mandates drinks containing a certain level of carcinogens come with a cancer warning label."[176]

Are we serious, here? Why are we knowingly poisoning each other?! The following is a list of items to avoid:

1. Artificial Colors. Artificial colors were originally derived from coal-tar dyes and petrochemicals. Coal-tar dyes are known cancer-causing agents, and over the last few decades, many of these dyes have been banned because of the fact that they have been deemed as such. "Today, the FDA (Food and Drug Administration) only allows ten colors in foods, four of which are restricted to specific uses."[177] This restriction definitely suggests that some risks remain, and in my personal opinion, we should all be wary. If you can buy food that has not been colored in any way, I would definitely suggest doing so. Better yet, make your own!

2. Artificial Flavors. The term "artificial flavors" refers to countless laboratory-created chemicals which have been designed to mimic the natural flavors found in nature.

A single artificial flavoring can be created from tons of individual chemical compounds, making it extremely difficult to narrow down a single harmful ingredient. New studies have suggested that artificial flavors can cause changes in an individual's behavior.[178] In fact, children who have been diagnosed with Attention Deficit Disorder (ADD) and autism have been found to be capable of much different behavior once additives, including artificial flavors, have been eliminated from their diets. Makes you wonder how many more needless prescriptions are out there . . .

3. Aspartame. This well-known sugar substitute is sold commercially under such names as Equal and NutraSweet. It's not recommended for pregnant women or children,[179] which really makes you think that no one should probably consume it, right? If you can't ingest it in a sensitive state for fear it could cause health concerns, then perhaps we should all be avoiding it.

4. Astaxanthin. Because close to 90% of salmon sold in grocery stores today come from fish farms and not an actual river, farmers add this chemical to the salmon to give it its desired pink color. Astaxanthin is produced from coal tar, the same carcinogen that food dyes are derived from.[180] Your farmed salmon is essentially being colored for you, with the added benefit of maybe contributing to your impending cancer. Salmon soufflé, anyone?

5. Benzoic Acid/Sodium Benzoate. These preservatives are often added to meat and meat-like products. They are used in many foods, including drinks, low-fat or low-sugar products, breakfast cereals and processed meats. Both of them are known to impair the normal functioning of digestive enzymes (not good news for digestive sufferers), and can cause migraine "headaches, stomach upset, asthma

attacks and hyperactivity in children."[181] (Yikes!) For anyone with a digestive issue, this one is definitely one to give up.

6. Butylated Hydroxyanisole (BHA) and Butylated Hydroxytoluene (BHT). These antioxidants are petroleum-based chemicals that are added to foods to prevent those foods from going bad. They are mostly found in snack food like crackers and potato chips, and meat products, such as sausages and dehydrated meats. The World Health Organization recognizes BHA a "possible human carcinogen."[182] Lovely.

7. Canthaxanthin. Egg producers use this chemical pigment to make egg yolks more yellow-colored. Although only teensy amounts are generally used, research has shown that this chemical has the ability to potentially cause damage to the retina of the eyes.[183] Yucky. This one may not affect digestion, but you kind of need your eyes, too . . . just sayin'.

8. Emulsifiers. These mixtures are used to extend the shelf life of bread products and allow liquids that wouldn't normally mix well to combine more smoothly. (Think of oil and water.) "Emulsifying agents used in foods include agar, albumin, alginates, casein, egg yolk, glycerol monostearate, xanthan gums, Irish moss, lecithin, and soaps."[184] Many of the ingredients just listed are very prevalent in processed foods. Just extra stuff that can cause allergic reactions that we do not need in our bodies.

9. High Fructose Corn Syrup. This super inexpensive sweetener helps maintain moisture while preserving freshness. The sheer quantity of this sweetener, used primarily in processed foods, is completely outstanding. Because it's a cheap way to get addictive sugar into cheap foods, it is everywhere. Consumption of this product in large quantities has been named a major factor in coronary heart disease (shocker!), which is the leading cause of death among men and women

both in Canada and the United States. It also raises cholesterol levels, while making blood cells more prone to clotting and greatly accelerating the aging process.[185] Stay away from this! It's gross, and almost always genetically modified.

10. Methylcyclopropene. This is a gas that is used to help preserve apples and pears (the more kid-friendly fruits), for around a year, and bananas for up to a month. Sulphur dioxide does the same thing when sprayed on grapes.[186] How many of you have bought apples in February and wondered how they look so good still? Ugghhh . . .

11. Monosodium Glutamate. (MSG) We all know this one, because of our awareness of it being commonly added to Chinese food to enhance flavor. MSG can be found in tons of processed products, not just chicken chow mien. MSG has been known to cause allergic responses, such as "tightening in the chest, headaches and a burning sensation in the neck and forearms."[187] (Getting something for nothing from something good for nothing . . .)

12. Olestra. You know it's bad when the FDA requires a warning label on foods containing this, right? But who ever sees the label? This totally fake fat was approved for use in snack foods several years ago, despite objections from dozens of researchers in food science. Olestra inhibits our ability to absorb good nutrients, and has also been known to cause "anal leakage" (ummm . . . hello!) and other gastrointestinal issues.[188] Wow. Talk about a bum deal.

13. Hydrogenated (or even "partially" hydrogenated) Oils. Hydrogenation occurs when oils are heated so that they become solids, and partial hydrogenation occurs when they become semi-solid, like butter. Examples are shortening and margarine. These oils are incredibly bad for you, because they become a denser form of fat than they were originally. They can be addictive, and definitely are known to lead to weight

problems, a slowed metabolism, diabetes, cancer and heart disease.[189] Seriously, if you are using margarine, throw it out. (Not that it will ever break down; it's also really bad for the environment, too.) Instead, if you really feel you must find a replacement, use Earth Balance Buttery Spread for a vegan option or old-school butter if you don't plan on giving up dairy.

14. Sodium Nitrite and Nitrate. These chemicals have been around for a long time, working to preserve meat. They are known to cause allergic reactions, and exacerbate cancer cell growth. These beauties are found in deli meats, hotdogs, bacon, breakfast sausages, etc.[190] In Kris Carr's bestselling book, *Crazy, Sexy, Diet*, she calls these meats "L&A" meats— meats that are made from lips and assholes.[191] Hungry? Remember: organic produce is made from water, sunshine, and love. A far cry from L&A. (Shudder . . .)

These fourteen ingredients are almost always present in any processed food, unless you pulled it off a shelf from the health food aisle. Even then, read the label to make sure. The less processed a food is, the less of these ingredients you will encounter. Hence, the "whole food" approach. When you eliminate processed foods, you automatically, without even thinking about it, eliminate loads of crazy chemicals from your diet.

Seeing red: I know a family whose daughter suddenly began suffering from an unknown allergy. Whatever she was eating was suddenly causing her face to break out in severe eczema, and subsequently made her miserable. She became very self-conscious and shy. It turned out that after extensive food eliminations and testing, which was done over the course of a few months using a trial and error method by her parents, the culprit turned out to be a very popular red food dye. Upon elimination of all foods with any dye, her face cleared up almost overnight. Crazy.

In Your Beauty Products

Don't forget: what you put on your skin in absorbed into your body; and although less directly, your digestive system too. The following statement was taken from the David Suzuki Foundation's website:[192]

"Some of the ingredients in beauty products aren't that pretty. U.S. researchers report that one in eight of the 82,000 ingredients used in personal care products are industrial chemicals, including carcinogens, pesticides, reproductive toxins, and hormone disruptors. Many products include plasticizers (chemicals that keep concrete soft), degreasers (used to get grime off auto parts), and surfactants (they reduce surface tension in water, like in paint and inks). Imagine what that does to your skin, and to the environment."[193]

The Dirty Dozen

The David Suzuki Foundation has been a respected charitable organization since 1990, and is a familiar name worldwide. The top goals of the foundation, as stated on their website, are to protect climate, transform Canadian economy, protect and reconnect with nature, and build community.[194]

Recently, the foundation surveyed Canadians to see how many of what they call the "Dirty Dozen" ingredients made appearances in their cosmetics. Apparently, that number is upwards of 80%. That means that four out of five beauty products that are on your shelves and in your drawers at home contain chemicals that have been proven toxic and carcinogenic.[195] You might want to grab a garbage bag . . . this applies to the United States, too.

The following twelve ingredients (all taken from www. davidsuzuki. org) are ones that should never make it into your home, especially in something that can be ingested or absorbed by you and your family. These substances are all capable of having effects on digestion, as well as other important body systems, whether by being absorbed through your largest organ (your skin), being ingested through food or water, or inhaled. Keep these away from you, and you will be healthier for it:

1. BHA and BHT. That's right—the same preservatives used in your food are used in beauty products, too. Gross. They are used mostly in lotions and cosmetics, are considered cancer-causing, and harmful to fish and other wildlife. Why do manufacturers think they could be okay for humans? They're not.

2. P-Phenylenediamine and colors listed as "CI" and followed by a number. These are coal tar dyes, and they possess the potential to cause cancer. They are also often contaminated with heavy metals, which can be absorbed through the skin and be toxic to your brain and central nervous system. An example would be FD&C Blue No. 1, or CI 75000.

3. DEA-related ingredients. These are used in foaming and creamy products, such as moisturizers, shaving creams, facial cleansers, and shampoos. They may be cancer-causing. Again, they are knowingly harmful to other wildlife, so wouldn't it be safe to assume that they would be harmful to us, too?

4. Dibutyl Phthalate. This ingredient is commonly used as a plasticizer in nail care products. They are suspected endocrine disruptors, and may be toxic to our reproductive systems. As far as our country's increasing infertility issues go, you have to wonder if chemicals might be a very strong contributor.

5. Formaldehyde-releasing preservatives. DMDM hydantoin, diazolidinyl urea, imidazolidinyl urea, methenamine and quarternium-15. They are used in a variety of cosmetics, and slowly release small amounts of the highly-toxic chemical formaldehyde. You know, the chemical commonly used to preserve corpses.

6. Parabens. Parabens are used in a variety of cosmetics as preservatives. They are often present in kids' bubble bath and shampoos. They are suspected endocrine disrupters and may

interfere with male reproductive functions. When I looked to see if my kids' shampoo and bath products had parabens in them, they all did. Five out of five. Needless to say, they were quickly disposed of, and replaced with ironically cleaner, organic products.

7. Fragrance. Present in almost all beauty products, soaps, laundry detergents, and cleaning products (sometimes even in those marked "unscented"), fragrances are highly toxic and can create allergic reactions such as a rash, itching, and sneezing. They are known to trigger asthma, which is why many workplaces now have a "no fragrance in the workplace" rule. Some fragrances are linked to cancer, and most are toxic to other forms of wildlife, also. If you are going to buy something that is scented, opt for an earth-friendly product that is scented with pure, organic essential oils.

8. PEG Compounds. These substances are cancer-causing, and are present in cosmetic cream bases and toothpaste. Ingredients with the letter combination "eth," such as polyethylene glycol, are often toxic ingredients and should be avoided.

9. Petrolatum. This toxic ingredient is used in hair products, lip balms, lipsticks, and moisturizers. By the name, you can probably deduce that it's a petroleum product. This particular one has been found to often be contaminated with polycyclic aromatic hydrocarbons, which can be cancer-causing.

10. Siloxanes. This substance is used in a wide variety of beauty products to help smooth, soften, and moisten. It's toxic to the reproductive system, and harmful to other wildlife and fish. Ingredients ending in "methicone" or "siloxane" are examples.

11. Sodium Laureth Sulfate. This ingredient is used in foaming cosmetics, such as shaving cream, foam bath, cleansers, and shampoos. It can be contaminated with dioxane, which

is cancer-causing. "Sodium Lauryl Sulphate" or "Sodium Laureth Sulphate" are two such offenders to watch out for.

12. Triclosan. This toxic substance is used in antibacterial beauty products, such as antiperspirants, face cleaners, and oral hygiene products. It is a suspected endocrine disruptor and can contribute to antibiotic resistance in bacteria. Again, like every other ingredient on this list of the Dirty Dozen, it is proven to be harmful to other wildlife.[196]

I was completely floored when I began comparing my products at home with this list. I have always been somewhat health conscious, and have always purchased what I thought were better quality products. Every single product that I possessed, at the time, had on average, four out of these twelve chemicals. Kid products are the worst, by the way. They are more colorful, more highly scented, and absolutely laden with chemicals off the Dirty Dozen list. Anyone else feel like we are being used as guinea pigs?

What about the *actual* guinea pigs?!

These substances are dangerous, and it's horrendous that they are permitted to be sold to unsuspecting consumers. If they can react with our endocrine, reproductive, and central nervous systems, why not our digestive systems? They just add to the high amount of garbage that our bodies are fighting to expel. Do yourself and your family a favor, and buy organic beauty products without these top twelve offenders. Try out some new products. Swap out your scented bubble bath for epsom salts or some pure essential oil. Get healthy in every aspect of your life, and you will feel better. I promise. By removing as many laboratory created, chemically derived, fake ingredients that we can from our lives, we can improve our health in countless ways, while making a statement to the producers of these products that they are completely unacceptable. The more we all lean towards demanding organic, clean products, the more those products will become available, and hopefully, the products that are chalk-full of carcinogens will slowly fall by the wayside and cease to be produced.

One of my favorite things to make on my own is a salt scrub. If you are into body exfoliation (which is great for improving circulation and sloughing off dead skin cells and toxins), stop buying commercial products. You can make your own with three ingredients: olive or jojoba oil, fine-grind epsom salt or medium-grind sea salt, and a few drops of pure, organic aromatherapy oil. I use lavender usually, but you can also try citrus, rosemary, peppermint, or whatever other scent you may enjoy. The ratio of oil to salt is up to you. I just take about a cup of salt, add oil and mix until I get the consistency that I like, and then add a few drops of lavender. Store the scrub in an airtight, glass container, like a used and washed jam jar. Voila! Easy body scrub that you can even make and give away as a gift. Just make sure that if you use epsom salt, that the salt is broken down a bit, and not in huge chunks.

> Itchy Issue: One of my children has skin reactions when he bathes in bubble baths, uses certain lotions, and when I wash his clothing in any detergent that has artificial fragrances. He breaks out in a rash, complains of itchiness, gets scaly skin, and sometimes becomes slightly asthmatic. If you or your kids have a similar problem, try eliminating the above ingredients from your life, and see what happens. It totally works wonders for my son.

Sugar: The Shady Lady

I like to call sugar "disease provoking." It is well known that the consumption of sugar wreaks havoc on our immune systems. Is the cold and flu season we all dread (especially if you have small children around) as much as an inevitability as we think? It coincides with Halloween, Christmas, New Years, and Valentine's Day, which all happen to be highly sugared-out holidays. Between the candy, chocolate, baking, and booze, our immune systems have no chance. Simple sugars (the kinds that are heavily processed and make our kids high, such as refined, white sugar and white flour), are so incredibly bad for us. They are highly addictive, and ultimately make us tired, cranky, and gain weight. Complex sugars that are present in whole grains and fruit provide long-lasting energy, and those are the sugars we should be indulging in.

Everybody knows that sugar has a bad reputation, because it is highly associated with diseases such as diabetes, candida (an overgrowth of yeast), and obesity. It is also known to completely disrupt the environment of your digestive system, by throwing off the balance of good-bad bacteria.

But what about sugar-like substances? Ingredients that are injected into food in order to account for its low levels of actual sugar when advertising its product as "sugar free," "low sugar," or "no added sugar?" I'm talking about the following culprits: "high fructose corn syrup, sucrose, glucose, fructose, lactose, maltose, dextrose, honey, corn syrup, invert sugar, invert sugar syrup, molasses, brown sugar, evaporated cane juice, sugar cane crystals, treacle, demerara sugar, fruit juice crystals, dehydrated fruit juice, corn sweetener, fruit juice concentrate, malt syrup, raw sugar, turbinado sugar, syrup, muscovado sugar, glucose syrup, barbados sugar, sorghum syrup, refiner's syrup, beet sugar, carob syrup, table sugar, malt, buttered syrup, maple syrup, rice syrup, agave nectar or syrup, powdered sugar, confectioner's sugar, corn syrup solids, d-mannose, sorbose, galactose, organic raw sugar, golden sugar, date sugar, castor sugar, golden syrup, and raisin syrup."[197]

Believe it or not, there are more of these. The problem is, the general public does not recognize these ingredients as sugar, so when examining a nutrition label, as we are all encouraged to do, clever marketers have substituted plain, old sugar for the above ingredients; many of which are chemically derived, which means that they are probably worse for you than the regular type of sugar we are all trying to avoid in the first place!

Are you frustrated yet? Your digestive system is.

The Glycemic Index: Choosing Your Sweets

The Glycemic Index (GI) ranks specific carbohydrates from zero to one hundred. This numerical value is based on how they affect your blood sugar levels after you eat them. Eating foods that have a high glycemic index number, such as soda, white flours, and candy, typically causes a major spike in blood sugar levels, which in turn results in a crazy energy crash. The goal of this plan is to eat carbohydrates that keep your blood sugar on a consistent level, therefore preventing spikes and crashes. You get more predictable energy this way, and you don't feel as hungry or desperate to eat at any given time. (Generally, the higher the GI number, the harder it is for your body to try and process.) The following is a list of different sweeteners, and where they fall on the GI list, ranking from worst offenders to least:

1. Glucose: 96
2. Sucrose (white sugar): 64
3. Brown sugar: 64
4. High fructose corn syrup: 62 (Sooo processed - don't ever eat this stuff!)
5. Evaporated cane juice: 55
6. Black strap molasses: 55
7. Maple syrup: 54
8. Lactose: 46 (The sugar in cow's milk)
9. Sugar cane juice: 43
10. Barley malt syrup: 42
11. Raw honey: 30
12. Brown rice syrup: 25 (This is great to bake with)
13. Fructose: 22 (Fruit)

14. Agave syrup: 15 (Great for drizzling on pancakes or over oatmeal)
15. Stevia: 1

Try and substitute refined, white sugar for something like brown rice syrup or agave syrup. They are lower on the glycemic index, and won't make your body work overtime.

The Past and the Present: What has Changed?

On several different occasions, I've had an acquaintance or two feel the need to point out to me that human beings have always eaten meat, and we are now unhealthier than ever before, in the midst of the current "health movement." In other words, there must be a correlation between the recently increased interest in health (in which a vegetarian diet has increasingly become more common), and the higher rates of disease than ever before.

Well, there is.

Only a hundred years ago, humans were dying for much different reasons. Things like bacterial infections, substandard hygiene, lack of antibiotics, childbirth complications, and diseases that are now preventable due to routine immunizations, were a few common ways to bite the dust. In present-day USA, none of these reasons are common anymore. The leading cause of death today is heart disease, something that can easily be traced back to our dietary choices. High blood pressure, high cholesterol, and obesity are all strong indicators of imminent heart disease. What do we do to lower those numbers? Eat less animal products (less saturated fat), and more vegetables. This super simple tweak would make huge strides in the direction of better health.

Back in the day (I'm still talking a hundred years ago; circa 1914), people grew their own vegetables, raised and slaughtered their own pigs, milked their own cows, and collected eggs from their own hens. The food was local, fresh, and free of today's antibiotics, hormones, GMOs, pesticides and herbicides. In other words, the chemical cocktail of today's food was non-existent, and so the quality was comparatively outstanding. The portions were also much smaller. These people had diets that were not primarily composed of processed foods, soda, fast food, bleached flour, or foods heavily laden with refined sugar and table salt. Of course they were healthier!

Today, our food rarely originates from the same cities we reside in, and an apple infused with pesticides and harvested two seasons ago is made far more available to us than an organic one, grown in our neighbourhoods, and harvested last week. That's messed up!

In the past, people used to work long, hard days on their own land, or land that was at least very close by. They used to do an incredible amount of manual labour, walk a lot more, and spend way more time outdoors. In comparison, in 2009, Americans commuted an average of fifty minutes a day.[198] We currently watch an average of four hours of television a day.[199] That amounts to about five hours a day sitting on our butts, not to mention those who sit for their forty-hour-a-week jobs, or actually take time to sit and eat dinner.

The quality of our food and the amount of activity we do is diminishing, and so is our health. We need to remember that although food keeps us alive, it's the *quality* of our food that determines for how long. It's not the current interest in health that is responsible for the record-breaking amount of disease that Americans and Canadians are enduring; it's the terrible quality of our food. Inadequate nutrition is the absolute largest factor in digestive disease and despair.

Did you know that under the current national food guidelines, a growing adolescent could meet all the recommended standards for healthy food intake, and still get away with eating sugary cereals, fast food, sodas, fried chicken, and potato chips every day? No wonder there is such a need for change in today's school cafeterias! We are feeding our kids terrible quality food, with almost no nutritional value. Eating like this on a regular basis means that our children will grow up obese, and continue this horrendous cycle with their own children. Our nation's wee ones are now being diagnosed on a regular basis with adult-onset diabetes.[200]

In Michael Pollan's book, *In Defense of Food*, he recommends that if your great-grandmother can't identify what something is at the grocery store, then leave it there.[201] If she gets a confused look on her face while staring at gelatinous treats, processed fruit snacks or canned meat, we need to take that as a sign. We have really only been experimenting with this type of food for a few decades, and so far, the results don't look good.

It's food that directly affects the state of our digestion. If you are experiencing digestive unease, you need to examine the type of fuel that your body is being expected to run on, and adjust the quality of that fuel accordingly. Putting sugary cereals, fast food, sodas, fried chicken, and potato chips into our body and expecting it to perform, is like diluting your gasoline with a higher and higher percentage of water every time you fill up. You might not see the effects right away, but eventually, your vehicle's going to stop working, and it might be too late to simply replace a few parts.

Question: What percentage of your pantry, refrigerator and freezer hold processed, sugary, nutritionally dead foods? What is the ratio of these items to real, whole foods that you think would be acceptable? If your kitchen does not reflect your ideal ratio, then tweak, baby, *tweak*!

Part Two

The How (The Plan)

Y ou've made it to part two; the heavy part is over. (Whew!) Learning the awful truths about your favorite foods can be disheartening, to say the least. Well, the lecture is done; time to move on. In the second half of the book, we'll focus on resolution instead of problems, so grab a highlighter or a pen and paper, and get ready to make some happy healthy notes. You'll discover some pretty fabulous solutions for greatly improving digestion as well as your overall health, including all things food. (And I'm talking about *good* food . . .)

Chapter 9

Get Wet!

pH stands for "potential of hydrogen," and its scale measures from pH 1 (very acidic), to pH 14 (very alkaline). In order to maintain homeostasis in the body, the pH of our blood is strictly regulated by a complex system that is always trying to maintain a pH range of approximately 7.15 to 7.25, which is slightly alkaline. The pH levels of our internal fluids affect every living cell in our bodies. If our bodies are too acidic (a pH level of less than 7), it can lead to devastating effects on our health, and therefore hinder disease prevention. An acidic pH level can create a breeding ground for which certain diseases (like cancer) can thrive.[202] It's just not possible to be healthy when the body is in a chronic state of acidosis. Therefore, if we want to maintain total body health, we need to make certain that our bodies stay slightly alkaline. The University of Tennessee sums this process up nicely:

". . . because water is the universal solvent for all life, it is important to know how its chemical properties can affect cells. One of the most important characterizations of a biological fluid is its pH. The concentration of hydrogen and hydroxide ions in an aqueous solution can greatly affect both the structure and chemical reactivity of cellular molecules. Cells . . . must maintain an appropriate pH in order to function optimally. Additionally, dramatic shifts in pH can play a role in controlling cellular activities such as egg division after fertilization. Consequently, cells must work constantly to maintain an acid-base balance. At the appropriate pH and concentration, buffers can be highly important in maintaining pH by preventing drastic changes."[203]

Most of the water that comes out of our taps here in North America is slightly acidic, usually somewhere around 6.5–7, and contains chlorine with the good intention to kill harmful bacteria. The pH of bottled water typically ranges from 3–8,[204] and is usually equivalent to most North American tap waters. (More on this in a minute . . .) In fact, almost all of the water we drink is acidic, when we need it to actually be slightly alkaline (as well as chlorine free and mineral rich) in order to hydrate our bodies to have optimal cell functioning.

The very best solution is to filter your own water. You can do this with a commercial filter, by owning a refrigerator with its own filtration system, or by installing a filtration system directly into your kitchen faucet.

It's also very important to recognize that what we eat directly affects our body's pH level. Essentially, foods that are acidic include all animal proteins and fats, alcohol, caffeine, refined sugars, and synthetic chemicals that are added to our food. Foods that promote alkalinity within the body are plant-based foods; mainly green, leafy vegetables. Remember, the idea is not to eat only alkaline foods, it is to make sure that there is a balance, and that the scales are tipped slightly in the direction of alkalinity. That means consuming mostly plant-based foods, and only eating acidic-forming foods in moderation.

"We have become too full of acid and, as a
result, are experiencing a wide range of diseases
that flourish in the acid medium."[205]
—Dr. Mary Ruth Swope, advocate for nutrition[206]

Alkaline Forming Foods

VEGETABLES
Alfalfa
Asparagus
Barley Grass
Beets
Broccoli
Brussel sprouts
Cabbage
Carrot
Cauliflower
Celery
Chard
Chlorella
Collard Greens
Cucumber
Dandelions
Dulce
Edible Flowers
Eggplant
Fermented Veggies
Garlic
Kale
Kohlrabi
Lettuce
Mushrooms
Mustard Greens
Nightshade
Onions
Parsnips (high glycemic)
Peas
Peppers
Pumpkin
Rutabaga
Sea Veggies
Spirulina
Sprouts
Squashes
Veggies
Watercress
Wheat Grass
Wild Greens

FRUITS
All Berries
Apple
Apricot
Avocado
Banana (high
glycemic)
Cantaloupe
Cherries
Currants
Dates/Figs
Grapes
Grapefruit
Lime
Honeydew Melon
Nectarine
Orange
Lemon
Peach
Pear
Pineapple
Tangerine
Tomato
Tropical Fruits
Watermelon

PROTEIN
Almonds
Chestnuts
Chicken Breast
Cottage Cheese
Eggs (poached)
Flax Seeds
Millet
Nuts
Powder
Pumpkin Seeds
Sprouted Seeds
Squash Seeds
Sunflower Seeds
Tempeh (fermented)
Tofu (fermented)
Whey Protein
Yogurt

OTHER
Alkaline Antioxidant
Apple Cider Vinegar
Banchi Tea
Bee Pollen
Dandelion Tea
Fresh Fruit Juice
Ginseng Tea
Green Juices
Green Tea
Herbal Tea
Kombucha
Lecithin Granules
Mineral Water
Organic Milk
(unpasteurized)
Probiotic Cultures
Veggies Juices
Water

SWEETENERS
Ki Sweet
Stevia

SPICES/SEASONINGS
All Herbs
Chili Pepper
Cinnamon
Curry
Ginger
Miso
Mustard
Sea Salt
Tamari

ORIENTAL VEGETABLES
Daikon
Dandelion Root
Kombu
Maitake
Nori
Reishi
Sea Veggies
Shitake
Umeboshi
Wakame

Acid Forming Foods

FATS & OILS	NUTS & BUTTERS	DRUGS & CHEMICALS
Avocado Oil	Brazil Nuts	Aspartame
Canola Oil	Cashews	Chemicals
Corn Oil	Peanut Butter	Drugs,
Flax Oil	Peanuts	Drugs, Medicinal
Hemp Seed Oil	Pecans	Herbicides
Lard	Tahini	Pesticides
Olive Oil	Walnuts	Psychedelic
Safflower Oil		
Sesame Oil	**ANIMAL PROTEIN**	**ALCOHOL**
Sunflower Oil	Beef	Beer
	Carp	Hard Liquor
FRUITS	Clams	Spirits
Cranberries	Fish	Wine
	Lamb	
GRAINS	Lobster	**BEANS & LEGUMES**
Amaranth	Mussels	Almond Milk
Barley	Oyster	Black Beans
Buckwheat	Pork	Chick Peas
Corn	Rabbit	Green Peas
Flour	Salmon	Kidney Beans
Hemp Seed	Scallops	Lentils
Kamut	Shrimp	Lima Beans
Oats (rolled)	Tuna	Pinto Beans
Quinoa	Turkey	Red Beans
Rice (all)	Venison	Rice Milk
Rice Cakes		Soy Beans
Rye	**PASTA (WHITE)**	Soy Milk
Spelt	Macaroni	White Beans
Wheat	Noodles	
Wheat Cakes	Spaghetti	
DAIRY	**OTHER**	
Butter	Distilled	
Cheese,	Potatoes	
Cheese, Cow	Vinegar	
Cheese, Goat	Wheat Germ	
Cheese, Sheep		
Milk		
Processed		

Another great way to balance your pH is to cut down on items that provide you no nutritional value, since most of these things are acidic. This list includes such items as sugar and processed food.

Kick these nasties to the curb! (To find out your pH level, contact your local naturopath or purchase a kit from a health-food store.)

We Are a Dehydration Nation

We can last weeks without food, but mere days without water. Water is vital for forming the foundation for blood, urine, digestive juices, and perspiration. The water content of your body is broken down the following way in these examples:

- Approximately 83% of blood is made up of water
- Approximately 75% of lean muscle (including brain tissue) is made up of water
- Approximately 10% of fat is water
- Approximately 22% of bone content is water[207]

Since your body is not capable of storing water for very long, it needs a fresh, new supply every day to account for losses, and needs to be replaced through what we eat and drink. The quality of our decisions affects how well this process works. Since foods provide only about one litre of fluid and the remainder must be obtained from what you drink, your choices in this matter are crucial. Some drinks are far more hydrating than others, so try and choose wisely.

Aside from water, coconut water is definitely my very favorite hydrating bevy. It possesses very few calories, and contains five different electrolytes for efficient hydration, making it the best-ever sports drink. My favorite brand of coconut water is O.N.E. This is not to imply that if you drink coconut water, that you don't need conventional water; regular, no-frills water is incredibly important to healing and rejuvenation of the entire body, and is absolutely required for proper digestion.

These are some things that water is needed for most:

- It aids digestion and prevents constipation
- It keeps your blood thin enough to flow through your blood vessels

- It helps to eliminate toxins
- Water regulates your body temperature by controlling perspiration
- It keeps mucous membranes moist, and lubricates joints
- It helps your bladder clear out bacteria
- It aids in maintaining the health and optimum function of every single cell in your body
- Water carries nutrients and oxygen to your cells[208]

If you are chronically dehydrated, you inadvertently increase your risk of developing kidney stones, constipation, urinary tract infections, and certain cancers.[209] Also, chronic dehydration has been linked to obesity, dwindling mental and physical performance, and decreased salivary gland function. Not a great prognosis for something as easily solvable as throwing back a few glasses of water each and every day.

If you are wondering if you might be dehydrated, check yourself for the following symptoms: headaches, migraines, lethargy, weakness, irritability, dry or cracked lips, dark-colored urine, and thick or foamy saliva. These are all signs of a body that is crying out for some liquid gold, stat!

We all know that drinking water is good for us. So, why does it seem that it is so difficult for so many people? I am willing to bet that most people living in North America drink less than sixteen ounces of water a day. Our bodies are made up of 60–70% water, depending on our age and the body part. (Example: babies are composed of more water than adults, and adult brains have more water than other adult body parts.) Water helps us stay hydrated in order to eliminate toxins through our urine and perspiration. It helps us keep cool, and our digestive tracts run smoothly. It keeps our skin clear and our other organs happy; particularly the liver and kidneys, which do most of our detoxifying for us.

I cannot stress enough how important water is. My challenge to you is to record for a week how many eight ounce glasses of water a day you drink. I'm not talking about juice, iced tea, coffee, alcohol, or pop. I'm talking straight-up water, or herbal tea (non-caffeinated). Hint: your daily total should reach around eight, and should be consumed at room temperature.

> Watered down results: try not to consume fluids while you eat. It interferes with proper digestion by diluting our stomach acid, which is responsible for digesting our food. If you have a hard time with digestion, do your stomach a favor and don't eat and drink at the same time.

If you are one to pound back the coffee, soda, black or green tea, and/or alcohol and forgo water, then you would still be dehydrated, despite consuming a ton of beverages throughout the day. Between our obsessions with sun tanning and chronically dehydrating ourselves, we're turning transforming ourselves into giant prunes. Ew!

If you feel you might benefit from some hardcore, cosmetic reasons to consume more water, then drink this up: regularly providing yourself with adequate amounts of water actually sends a signal to the body telling it that you are not in danger of dehydration, and that your body can afford to let go some of its extra fluid. Water retention is often to blame for puffy eyes and skin, particularly in the face, neck, hands, and feet. If you feel that your appearance could improve by losing some of this puffiness, then one of the easiest things you can do is to step up the water intake. It will flush out all of that fluid that your body has been holding onto, and the result will be a smoother, slimmer, more hydrated appearance. Drinking oodles of water also helps with acne and dry skin, since the skin is your largest organ, and water helps your organs to re-hydrate and detoxify. Also, many doctors will agree that increased water intake helps to reduce the appearance of cellulite. Why pay for lipo? Go get your drink on! (Water, that is . . .)

The other sneaky substance that we should be aware of that greatly contributes to dehydration is salt. Salt is over-abundantly in everything, from canned soups to frozen entrees. Commonly listed as sodium chloride or sodium benzoate, many consumers don't realize that this ingredient is actually table salt. Try purchasing products that don't have added salt, and that will lend a small hand in the hydration department. Also, if you are in the habit of adding salt to recipes, try sprinkling a little bit on *after* cooking your meal, not *while* cooking your meal. Research shows that even if you use salt in your cooking, you will probably still add more salt to it once the food is plated. Skip the salt in the middle, and just add it if you must at the end. Lastly, use sea salt instead of table salt, the latter of which is very refined.

On the digestion front, increasing your water intake could be the best thing you can do to help a lazy, temperamental bowel. If you have issues with constipation or hard stools, then a little extra water would definitely work wonders for you. In fact, drinking an eight ounce glass of warm water infused with a squeeze of lemon first thing upon waking is the very best way to stimulate your bowels and get an early start to your day. (Especially if you sprinkle some cayenne pepper in there.)

If you are suffering on the other end of the spectrum, and experience a lot of diarrhea, then water is equally important to rehydrate your body after the sudden loss of so much fluid. If this is the case for you, try adding a pinch of sea salt to the water, or try your hand at coconut water. It will replace lost electrolytes that your body desperately needs.

An important note on bottled water: although tap water may contain high levels of chlorine and other nasties, it is still strictly regulated. Bottled water is not. Bottled water often comes from municipal taps, and once it's stored in packaging that contains harmful chemicals such as BPA (Bisphenol A) and PET (polyethylene terephthalate), the water becomes contaminated with those chemicals, *as well* as the original levels of chlorine. Bottled water is a little scary. Again, your best bet is to have a filtration device installed in your home for tap water.

Pause your reading of this book for a minute, and go drink a glass of water. (Hopefully filtered, so it has a good pH level . . .)

Question: How many glasses of water do you drink in a day? If you don't think you drink enough, what will you do to ensure proper hydration?

Highlight: Marie's Story

I have fibromyalgia. For those who don't know what fibromyalgia is, it is a medical disorder that is characterized by chronic, widespread pain and allodynia, a heightened and painful response to pressure. The pain affects muscles, tendons and joints, as well as causes stiffness. Chronic fatigue, restless leg syndrome, and a long list of other symptoms make this disorder very uncomfortable to live with. It is also aggravated by noise, weather change and emotional stress.

My journey with this disorder began in 2006 when I was diagnosed. Over the space of six years my condition worsened, until at the beginning of 2012, when I was at the end of my tether with it. My pain had become unbearable most days. Sometimes I would shut myself in the bathroom, away from my husband and just sob, as I was finding it harder and harder to cope from day to day. Not being able to sleep properly at night was not helping, either. To add misery to the pain, I also found that certain foods I ate seemed to make it worse. Because of stiffness, it was becoming increasingly difficult to climb stairs or walk long distances, especially if the ground wasn't flat. Travelling long distances in a car or on a plane was almost unbearable. The day to day chores became harder. By lunch time most days I was exhausted and just wanted to sleep.

On the first day of February 2012, I decided that I had nothing to lose by trying a total change in the way I eat. I went vegan . . . I didn't try easing myself into it as I knew from past efforts to eat differently that it wouldn't work for me. It was all or nothing. I also went gluten and wheat free, as both of these have proved countless times to makes my pain worse.

I have been on this new way of eating for almost ten months and I can only describe how I feel as a miracle.

After just one week of eating this way I started noticing changes in how I felt. Pain started to disappear, sleep patterns improved, and I had energy to burn. Now I find I can run up and down three flights of stairs to our condo, whereas just before I had started this eating plan, my husband had decided that we should move into a building that had an elevator or at least live at ground level. Travelling is no longer a nightmare. I can walk for miles, up and down hills.

I have no intention to ever eat meat or any animal by-products again. My diet is full of fresh fruit and vegetables, beans, legumes, nuts, lentils and whole grains. I also take a supplement to cover my B vitamins.

I am living proof that what we eat affects our health.

Chapter 10

Serious Solutions for Happy Digestion

Before we get started with this chapter, here's the deal: this book is not really about a diet, so let's not focus on that particular word. When I hear the word *diet* I envision calorie counting, food weighing, and being hungry all the time. Well, that's not how I roll!

This book is about changing your life, one lifestyle choice at a time. You need to ask yourself, "Am I willing to work at this? Do I want to ditch this poor digestive crap? Do I want to feel good, and maintain a good, healthy body weight? Do I want to sleep better, breathe deeper, and think more clearly?" If your answer is a resounding "Yes, please!", then you are looking for a solid foundation of wellness: a full-on platform, which is where this book comes in. Why feel good, when you can feel awesome?

Not just about food, the decision to make a dramatic change in one's health is about tapping into another world, one of being closer to the earth, closer to others, and above all, closer to yourself. It's about finding the foods that feed your soul, not just your appetite. It's about introducing practices into your daily routine that strengthen you from the inside out, physically, emotionally, and spiritually. It's pretty empowering! The following are some basic instructions to help you build your perfect happy-gut platform:

Read the Ingredients List

Don't worry. I'm not suggesting that you try to calculate how much protein versus carbohydrates a food should contain, or how many calories you should be consuming on a daily basis. That's the great thing about eating well; you don't have to care about calories or carbohydrates. I'm not even suggesting that you begin deciphering the nutrition labels. I'm talking about actually reading the list of ingredients, observing how many there are, and noticing the ones you've never heard of before. Also, make sure to be on the look-out for a few specific ones. Here are some general rules to follow when choosing your food:

1. Don't buy anything with a long list of ingredients. The fewer the better. Less ingredients means less processed. You'd be amazed at the difference in ingredients for the same type of food. For example, some yogurts on the market have about twenty-five ingredients in them; some have three. If you cannot live without yogurt, buy the brand that has three. (Liberté Organic Plain is one example.)

2. Don't buy anything that has sugar listed in the first three ingredients. Remember that sugar comes in a plenitude of forms, with many, many different names. Try and memorize the list before shopping. Who am I kidding? Take the list with you! You will cut out an outstanding amount of sugar from your diet this way. Naturally occurring sugars, such as sugar that is found in fruit (fructose) is okay. (For example, homemade fruit leather is high in sugar, but it all comes from the fruit itself.)

3. Ingredients that are nutritionally unnecessary should be avoided. This includes any preservative, artificial flavor

or color, gelatine, and sugar (especially high fructose corn syrup, which is extremely processed and more often than not, genetically modified).

4. Be wary about anything that you cannot pronounce. These ingredients are lab-created, and not food. As I have read many times in previous books on this topic, you should not have to have a chemistry degree to know what's in your food.

5. Know that food manufacturers are sneaky. "Apple drink" sounds like apple juice, but it's not. "Enriched flour" sounds like it could mean "whole grains," but in fact is stripped of any nutrients whatsoever. Organic cane sugar might sound like a great health alternative, but it is still sugar. Remember that just because something has an earthy sounding name, does not mean it's from the earth. A lot of these fancy names are from the lab; don't judge a food by its cover!

6. Shop the perimeter of the grocery store. It's actually better if you can buy a large percentage of your food from farmer's markets, but if you're at the grocery store, the best products are found on the outside edge of the building. The entire middle section is what I call the "processed pit," and should be avoided if you can help it. (Except the health food aisle.) Your grocery cart should contain approximately 50% whole grains, nuts, seeds, and beans, 40% fruits and vegetables, and about 10% of your favorite less-processed foods, like dried fruit, organic soups, organic dark chocolate, olives, hummus, or yummy, crispy, grainy crackers. We're only human; we need us some goodies!

Organics

"I don't care about spots on my apples, leave me the birds and the bees . . . "[210]

—Joni Mitchell

It took me years to fully understand the deal with organics. Even a couple of years ago, I was only half convinced. I didn't like that the products were sometimes significantly more expensive (sometimes $1.99 per pound for apples versus $.99), and I didn't understand what that difference meant to the health of my tummy, and to my family. Now I do.

Certified organic products contain no toxic chemicals, herbicides, pesticides, artificial colors or flavors, and certainly no antibiotics, growth hormones or genetically modified ingredients. They are more expensive because they are more difficult, and generally more expensive to produce. Because organic vegetable farmers do not use pesticides, they must keep little critters and hungry bugs away using different methods, which can be labour intensive and definitely requires more creativity in the prevention department. In other words, it's way more difficult to grow organically than to grow conventionally. However, it is much better for the consumer, and for the environment. Chemicals used

Does size really matter? Often when you purchase organic fruit and vegetables, they are smaller than non-organic pieces of produce. I assumed that this was a sign of no chemical intervention. A couple of year ago, my neighbour, whose parents have an enormous organic vegetable garden, brought me some produce that would go to waste if not dispersed. There were two big bags of endive, beets, and carrots, and they were *giant!* These carrots and beets were so massive, that I could juice one carrot and get the same amount of juice that I usually received from about four. It was pretty sweet.

to kill bugs and weeds, deter rodents, and prematurely ripen fruit get absorbed into the ground, and eventually make their way to water. Once there, they affect fish and other living things that are definitely *not* trying to eat our apples. When we spray, we inevitably (though unintentionally) affect not only our produce, but also other innocent life.

In regards to food animals, raising cattle (and other animals) organically means that those cows can only consume organic feed, and can only live in organic spaces. This goes as far as being contained in pasture with non-treated wooden fence posts. It also means no herbicides, pesticides, or genetically altered materials have ever entered their bodies. Further, they have never been treated with an antibiotic, which means that their living conditions are usually much better than that of the millions of cattle raised by today's more common practices. (They aren't knee-deep in their own waste, which is often the cause for antibiotics in the first place.) Also, they have never been fed growth hormones. All of this care and attention generally means healthier cattle, which in turn produces more nutritious beef.

If the idea of paying more for organic products is still a deterrent for you, then consider that the entire operation surrounding the use of pesticides and herbicides is expensive business. If everyone (or even a larger percentage of us) decided to go the organic route, we would be saving an astronomical amount of money that would otherwise be fed into the business of producing harmful chemicals and less nutritious food. We have the power to vote with our dollar for better food. We should let the food industry know what we think of their products by whether or not we choose to purchase them. If we continue to buy sub-par food, more will be produced because it shows that there is a market for it. Likewise, by purchasing good quality, highly nutritious food, it will show that there is a growing demand for the good stuff!

Shopping organic means knowing that what you are about to eat is chemical, GMO, antibiotic, and hormone free. Who knows how the incredible overabundance of these "revolutionary products" are affecting your digestive system, but they undoubtedly are. If you want to be certain that chemical cocktails remain out of your lunch, and in turn, out of your digestive tract, then you need to go for the Big O . . .

Here are ten reasons why you should consider eating organically, all of which are undisputedly related to your health. This compilation was taken directly from Green Earth Organics,[211] and it makes a solid case for the many benefits of adopting an organic diet:

1. "Protect future generations. Children receive four times the exposure than an adult to at least eight widely used cancer-causing pesticides in food. The food choice you make now will impact your child's health in the future.

2. Prevent soil erosion. The Soil Conservation Service Estimates that more than three billion tons of topsoil are eroded from the United States croplands each year. That means soil is eroding seven times faster than it is built up naturally. Soil is the foundation of the food chain in organic farming. But in conventional farming the soil is used more as a medium for holding plants in a vertical position so they can be chemically fertilized. As a result, American and Canadian farms are suffering from the worst soil erosion in history. (Poor soil quality directly contributes to poor produce quality.)

3. Protect water quality. Water makes up two-thirds of our body mass and covers three-fourths of the planet. Despite its importance, the Environmental Protection Agency (EPA) estimates pesticides (some cancer-causing) contaminate the ground water in thirty-eight states, polluting the primary source of drinking water for more than half the country's population.

4. Save energy. Farms have changed drastically in the last three generations, from the family based small businesses dependent on human energy to large scale factory farms highly dependent on fossil fuels. Modern farming methods use more

petroleum than any other single industry, consuming 12% of the country's total energy supply. More energy is now used to produce synthetic fertilizers than to till, cultivate, and harvest all the crops in the United States. Organic farming is still mainly based on labour-intensive practices, such as weeding by hand and using green manures and crop covers rather than synthetic inputs. Organic produce also tends to travel a shorter distance from the farm to your plate.

5. Keep chemicals off your plate. Many pesticides approved for use by the EPA were registered before extensive research linking these chemicals to cancer and other diseases had been established. Now the EPA considers that 60% of all herbicides, 90% of all fungicides and 30% insecticides are carcinogenic. A 1987 National Academy of Sciences report estimate that pesticides might cause an extra 1.4 million cancer cases among Americans over their lifetimes. The bottom line is that pesticides are poisons designed to kill living organisms, and can also be harmful to humans. In addition to cancer, pesticides are implicated in birth defects, nerve damage and genetic mutation.

6. Protect farm workers' health. A National Cancer Institute study found that farmers exposed to herbicides had a greater factor of six, than non-farmers of contracting cancer. In California, reported pesticide poisonings among farm workers have risen an average of 14% a year since 1973, and doubled between 1975 and 1985. Field workers suffer the highest rates of occupational illness in the state. Farm workers health also is a serious problem in developing nations, where pesticides can be poorly regulated. An estimated 1 million people are poisoned annually by pesticides. Several of the pesticides banned from use in the United States are still manufactured here for export to other countries.

7. Help small farmers. Although more and more large scale farms are making the conversion to organic practices, most organic farms are small independently owned and operated family farms of less than one hundred acres. It's estimated that the United States has lost more than 650,000 family farms in the past decade. With the US Department of Agriculture predicting that half of this country's farm production will come from 1% of farms by the year 2000. Organic farming could become one of the few hopes left for family farms.

8. Support a true economy. Although organic food might seem more expensive than conventional foods, conventional food prices do not reflect hidden cost borne by taxpayers, including nearly $74 billion in federal subsidies in 1988. Other hidden costs include pesticide regulation and testing, hazardous waste disposal and clean up, and environmental damage.

9. Promote biodiversity. Mono cropping is the practice of planting large plots of land with the same crop year after year. While this approach tripled farm production between 1950 and 1970, the lack of natural diversity of plant life has left the soil lacking in natural minerals and nutrients. To replace the nutrients, chemical fertilizers are used, often in increasing amounts.

10. Taste better flavor. There's a good reason many chefs use organic foods in their recipes. They taste better. Organic farming starts with the nutrients of the soil which eventually leads to the nourishment of the plant and ultimately our palates."[212]

It's also important to understand that for a farm to be certified organic, it must adhere to incredibly strict guidelines that require extra time, patience and incredible expense to attain. Farmers who choose to go the organic route, whether their fare may be produce or animal products, definitely deserve special accolades.

The Dirty Dozen of Pesticide-Ridden Produce (Top twelve foods to always buy organic)[213]

1. Peaches	7. Cherries
2. Apples	8. Pears
3. Bell Peppers	9. Grapes
4. Celery	10. Spinach
5. Nectarines	11. Lettuce
6. Strawberries	12. Potatoes

The Consistently Clean List (Top twelve foods that test relatively clean for pesticides)[214]

1. Onions	7. Sweet Peas
2. Avocado	8. Kiwis
3. Sweet Corn	9. Bananas
4. Pineapples	10. Cabbage
5. Mangoes	11. Broccoli
6. Asparagus	12. Papaya

Superfoods

You've probably heard the term *superfood* before. It refers to a variety of foods, all plant-based, that hold extraordinary nutritional value. The "top ten superfoods" seem to be constantly changing, but not out of the whole food, plant-based realm. The following list is my own personal compilation of superfoods— what I consider to be nutritionally invaluable, and the ones I have at my disposal at all times. Some I use on a weekly basis, others I use daily.

1. Berries. Super full of antioxidants, berries help to fight against diseases, such as cancer, Alzheimer's, and more. When they're in season (June–August), you can buy fresh berries by the flat from farmers' markets. Eat as much as you can fresh, and

freeze the rest for smoothies. In the off-season, you can buy organic, frozen berries for smoothies and baking.

2. Broccoli. Broccoli is super high in magnesium, calcium, potassium, and vitamin C. It contains high amounts of chlorophyll and fiber, and can be used in a variety of ways. I chow down on steamed broccoli about twice a week, and juice with it almost daily.

3. Chia seeds. These tiny seeds are super high in soluble fiber, omega 3 fatty acids, and protein. They lend fabulous energy and are quite effective when incorporated into weight-loss plans. I use chia seeds in smoothies and oatmeal almost daily.

4. Chlorella. Chlorella is a fresh-water algae. It is crazy high in chlorophyll and nucleic acids. It is also a complete protein, and contains vitamin B12, making it a veggie-lover's dream supplement. I use a powdered form of this sea green in smoothies (about one teaspoon of it), a couple of times throughout the week, and I also take it in pill form almost daily.

5. Ginger. Fresh ginger, in particular, can be a lifesaver for anyone with digestive issues. It is naturally anti-inflammatory, and relieves nausea and flatulence. It can be added to any juice or smoothie for a crazy flavor-changer, too. I juice with it often, almost daily.

6. Hemp. Legal to grow in Canada, but illegal to grow in the U.S., this protein-packed, environmentally sustainable superfood is extremely undervalued and underappreciated. It is composed of 35% protein, making it a fabulous alternate protein source for vegetarians. It also requires less water to grow than other plants, and less space. Hemp can be consumed either by eating the hemp hearts themselves, or in a hemp-based protein powder. I cook raw hemp hearts about twice a week, and use Vega hemp protein powder almost daily.

7. Kale. Kale is a nutritional superstar. It is extremely high in antioxidants, vitamins A, C and K, fiber, and is low in

calories. It is a cruciferous vegetable, like broccoli, and is teeming with chlorophyll. You can steam it, juice it, add it to soups and stews, make chips out of it, and more. Definitely add this one to your grocery list. I use kale about twice a week to make the kale chip recipe in chapter thirteen.

8. Quinoa. This South American grain is actually a seed, and is a complete protein. It's super versatile, and can be consumed in place of rice or millet. It is higher in calcium, phosphorus, magnesium, potassium, iron, copper, manganese, and zinc, and lower in sodium compared with wheat, barley and corn. I cook up a big batch of quinoa about once a week, and use it for a variety of different dishes.

9. Raw nuts. These gems are all freakin' fabulous! They are full of omega 6 fatty acids, and although high in calories, they are teeming with nutrients to include into your plant-based diet. I eat about ¼ cup of raw nuts on a daily basis, rotating through an assortment of almonds, pecans, walnuts, and hazelnuts.

10. Sea vegetables. Usually just called seaweed, sea vegetables are not usually part of the North American diet, but they should be. They veggies are incredibly nutritionally dense, packed with calcium, iron, chlorophyll, and naturally occurring electrolytes. Different types of sea vegetables are nori (I use this often), dulse, kelp, wakame, arame, agar, and kombu. I use nori about twice a week, and whenever I go to a Japanese restaurant, I order a wakame salad. Soooo yummy.

Eat the Rainbow

Did you know that the color of your produce is indicative of the healthful benefits that it contains? Vegetables rich in color are full of phytonutrients (plant nutrients), which are recently found to offer immense health benefits. There are many types of phytonutrients, including antioxidants, plant sterols, natural acids, and enzymes.[215]

Think about what you eat for dinner. If your average meal consists of fried chicken, mashed potatoes, gravy, and a processed, white bun, what colors are present? Brown and white? Your diet would be extremely lacking in vitamins and minerals, which are absolutely essential to not only digestive health, but your overall state of form and function. In order to benefit from all of nature's nutritional gifts, you must get used to eating the rainbow.

Red

Lycopene is a nutrient found in red fruits and vegetables, such as tomatoes, red bell peppers, pink grapefruit, cherries and watermelon. It is good for the skin, and is known to help prevent against certain cancers.[216]

Orange

Beta-Carotene is present in such foods as carrots, pumpkins, sweet potatoes, mangoes, cantaloupe and apricots. This well-known phytonutrient helps to improve cellular communication, and is great for protecting eyesight.[217]

Yellow

Yellow fruits and vegetables such as lemons, papaya, pineapple, nectarines, and peaches contain flavanoids and Vitamin C. Flavanoids possess anti-inflammatory properties, which is essential for digestive health. Vitamin C plays a huge role in protecting the body against infections by strengthening the immune system, which is also happy news.[218]

Green

Green bell peppers, honeydew melon, kiwi, green beans, avocados, spinach, and other leafy green vegetables are among the members of the green family that provides the plant nutrient lutein. Lutein protects the body against free radicals and macular degeneration. It also is great for the skin.[219]

Purple

Anthocyanins are highly concentrated in fruits and vegetables that are blue and purple, such as blueberries, blackberries, eggplant, plums, prunes, beets, red cabbage, purple grapes, and acai. They are strong antioxidants, and are fantastic for immune health, among other benefits.[220]

The Vegan Food Pyramid

We all remember the USDA food pyramid from our elementary school years, right? Beginning at the bottom, it recommended 6-10 serving of grains and cereals, then 3-5 servings of fruits and vegetables, then 2-3 servings of dairy, 2-3 servings of meat, poultry, or fish, and then finally it recommended that you only eat sweets, fats, and oils sparingly.

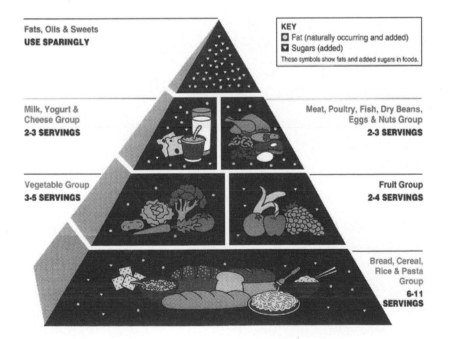

Well, out with the old, in with the new! The brand new 2011 "MyPlate" is the equivalent of the old-school food pyramid from the past. It almost divides veggies, fruit, meat, and grains into quarters, and then recommends dairy on the side. The serving suggestions appear to be somewhat equal, and I guess I would perceive it as this: 40% of your food intake should be produce (awesome), 35% should be "protein" and dairy (a little high), and 25% grains (a little low).

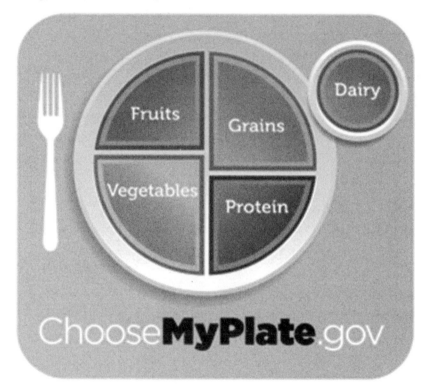

While I do have to give the government props for the larger percentage of fruits and veggies, and also for labelling the previous "meat and alternatives" category "protein," I still argue that 35% protein is completely unnecessary, and 25% grains is probably too little. Also, "whole grains" should be emphasized. With just "grains"

sitting there, alot of people might infer that a roll of saltines is just as good for you as a cup of quinoa (which, of course, it isn't).

Well, I have a better one for you, my friend. The Vegan Food Guide provides a good visual on how much of what foods you should be eating. If you decide to take the plunge and adopt a plant-based diet, this will serve you well as a great reference. Simply print one off the internet, and stick it on your refrigerator.

VEGAN FOOD GUIDE
DAILY PLAN FOR HEALTHY EATING

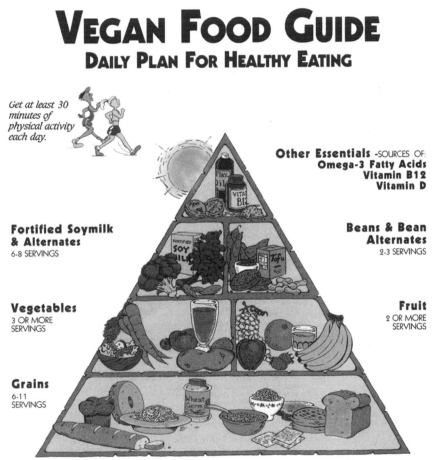

Get at least 30 minutes of physical activity each day.

Other Essentials -SOURCES OF:
Omega-3 Fatty Acids
Vitamin B12
Vitamin D

Fortified Soymilk & Alternates
6-8 SERVINGS

Beans & Bean Alternates
2-3 SERVINGS

Vegetables
3 OR MORE SERVINGS

Fruit
2 OR MORE SERVINGS

Grains
6-11 SERVINGS

Artwork by Dave Brousseau

Eat a variety of foods from each of the food groups.
Drink 6-8 glasses of water and/or other fluids each day.
Limit intake of concentrated fats, oils, and added sugars, if used.

"It is the position of the American Dietetic Association and Dieticians of Canada that appropriately planned vegetarian diets are healthful, nutritionally adequate, and provide health benefits in the prevention and treatment of certain diseases. Well-planned vegan and other types of vegetarian diets are appropriate for all stages of the life cycle, including during pregnancy, lactation, infancy, childhood, and adolescence. Vegetarian diets offer a number of nutritional benefits, including lower levels of saturated fat, cholesterol, and animal proteins, as well as higher levels of carbohydrates, fiber, magnesium, potassium, folate, and antioxidants, such as vitamins C and E and phytochemicals. Vegetarians have been reported to have lower body mass indices than non-vegetarians, as well as lower rates of death from ischemic heart disease; vegetarians also show lower blood cholesterol levels; lower blood pressure; and lower rates of hypertension, type 2 diabetes, and prostate and colon cancer."[221]

—Journal of the American Dietetic Association

Food Combining

If you have never heard of food combining, then your tummy is in for a treat. Theoretically, food combining makes digestion easier by only having to deal with specific types of food at any one time, depending on how long they plan on hanging out in your digestive system. For instance, fruit is digested the fastest; meat the slowest. This works for me, and it may also work for you.

Fruits should be eaten alone, or with each other. They digest so quickly (in most part because of the high sugar composition), that they are already semi-digested by the time they arrive in your stomach. If the fruits are combined with other foods, they will get trapped, and begin to rot and ferment, causing gas. Melons digest at an extremely speedy rate, so it's best to eat these alone.

Protein and starch don't mix very well. To digest proteins, your body needs an acidic base. An alkaline base is required in order to digest starches. Both proteins and starches combine well with veggies, but they do not combine very well with each other. In other words, my once-favorite snack of cheese and crackers is out. So is pizza, creamy pasta, grilled cheese sandwiches, etc. If you have a tough time with digestion of any kind, this one adjustment could really help you out.

Don't eat proteins and fats together. Fats inhibit digestion, and proteins take the longest to digest, so this can equal constipation. This is another reason to forgo meat. Red meat, especially, contains high amounts of protein and fat, so it's particularly difficult to digest.

This whole procedure sounds tedious, but I can personally assure you of its eventual simplicity. To sum up, proteins are great with veggies, starches are great with veggies, proteins and starches should not be combined, nor should protein and fats, and eat fruit by itself.

For the very best results, try to wait the following lengths of time between consuming foods that don't combine well:[222]

- Fruit needs two hours. (Melons take only fifteen minutes to digest; the rest of the fruit takes about an hour.)
- Starches need three hours. (They take approximately three hours to digest.)
- Proteins need four hours. (Plant-based protein takes about four hours; animal-based protein takes anywhere from eight hours for fish to seventy-two hours for beef to digest.)

If you notice that within an hour or so after eating that your stomach responds by bloating, cramping, and generally begins to feel inflamed, you should definitely try food combining. (Or ask yourself if you just ate some dairy . . . dairy causes stomach cramps, too.) Food combining is not difficult; it just takes a little practice, and it's completely worth it.

*It is important to note that although I've had positive personal experiences using this strategy, there is no reliable scientific evidence showing that food combining works. Just keepin' it real.

Buying Locally

In *The 100-Mile Diet*, by Vancouverites Alisa Smith and J.B. MacKinnon, they explain that the vast majority of the food that reaches plates in Canada (this also applies to the United States), has travelled an average of 1500 miles.[223] That means that although seriously delicious, those avocados from Mexico or bananas from Fiji are pretty old by the time they get eaten. Fruit and vegetables' nutrients begin to diminish the moment they are picked or harvested. The best way to take advantage of what a piece of produce has to offer is to eat it within a few days of it being plucked, or to freeze it right away. (A process termed "flash-frozen.") Other foods count, too. Try and purchase local eggs, bread, dairy, and other staple items. Before throwing something into your shopping cart, look at the label to figure out where it was produced. I was pretty excited to figure out that my very favorite bread (generally anything made from Silverhills Sprouted Bakery), is produced in the same city that I live in! By buying locally, you are sure to reap the benefits of better quality food, because it is still fresh, and spent far less time in transit. There are also other numerous advantages to local shopping:

Reduction of your ecological footprint is a great reason to try and stick to local foods. If that food you're holding has never seen a long-haul truck, cargo boat, train, or an airplane, then the amount of fuel you have saved by purchasing locally is outstanding. Supporting local economy is another great excuse to buy your apples from the farm down the road. Even though buying local is not always less expensive, it usually is. Most people wouldn't mind spending the extra few bucks' difference if it means supporting local farmers. In addition, buying local translates to better traceability of our food, which more and more consumers are beginning to realize is something that is important to them. Being connected to our food is special. Food keeps us alive, and determines our health. Knowing where it comes from and who it's produced by is both powerful and exciting.

Exploring the diversity of local produce is interesting, because eating locally also means eating seasonally. This is important, because our twenty-first century, on-demand lifestyles often exemplify the fact that we've collectively lost our knowledge regarding which season brings what food. Every fruit and vegetable has a season, and those products taste way better when they are in season, compared with when they aren't. Have you ever had watermelon and thought it wasn't very flavorful? What about strawberries? That was probably because they weren't in season. Eating in season is fun, and it's all local.

Being confident about the quality of your food is another pretty sweet by-product of purchasing local. You might have a pretty good idea about the ins and outs of your own country's laws regarding pesticides, herbicides, antibiotics, hormones, and genetically modified organisms, but do you know Japan's? I like feeling sure about what restrictions were imposed on the farmers who grew the pear that I am about to feed to my children. Do you know how mandarin oranges grow, or what might be used to modify them, preserve them, or enhance their color or flavor? Hmmm . . .

Fermenting Vegetables

Eating fermented vegetables once or twice a week can be one of the best things you can do for your overall health. Fermentation is a fabulous way to preserve good food, ensuring vitamin-rich nourishment all year long. It also floods the digestive system with beneficial microflora which can help keep your gut healthy and strong. Healthy bacterial cultures are also present in cultured or fermented vegetables. The more healthy microflora one keeps in one's gut, the more the body's receptors are blocked when exposed to dangerous viruses and bacteria, such as *Salmonella* or *Listeria*. Fermented vegetables are also high in natural antioxidants and benefit general health in many ways. Call your loveliest of friends, crack open a bottle of organic red wine, and have a fermenting party!

How to Ferment Vegetables

Step 1: Choose your veggies. Great vegetables to ferment include cabbage and/or cucumbers (the staples), and then bell peppers, radishes, beets, carrots, and onions. You can ferment any veggie, but these are the ones most people prefer to work with.

Step 2: Chop or grate them up into the desired size. I like to keep mine big enough to throw on burgers, sandwiches, and salads. Some people like to mince their veggies in a food processor, because the smaller the pieces, the faster they will ferment. Once chopped, throw them all in a 500 ml Mason jar. The veggies should reach to the top of the jar.

Step 3: Add your brine. The standard recommendation is one litre of fluid to two tablespoons of good quality sea salt. For a 500 ml jar, try adding half a tablespoon of sea salt to about one cup of filtered water. Mix well. Ensure that the salt has dissolved completely and then pour the brine into the jar, over the veggies. The liquid should fill the jar to the top, completely encapsulating the vegetables and ensuring even fermentation.

Step 4: Once all the veggies are submerged in the brine, cap the jar and keep on your counter in room temperature.

Step 5: The jar should remain there for about a week. Open the jar daily to release any pressure, and begin tasting your veggies around day five. Once you like the way it tastes, put the jar in your refrigerator to store. It can stay there until it's all gone . . . it's preserved!

Your newly pickled veggies will taste great on sandwiches, veggie burgers, or even just by themselves. Experiment!

Sprouting

There are many people who find that they have a tough time digesting grains, seeds, beans, and legumes. In fact, many of us avoid beans and legumes because of the gas produced by eating them, which can quickly turn into embarrassing flatulence episodes. (My worst nightmare scenario for this is a crowded, quiet yoga class!) The best way to curb this effect is by sprouting the grains, seeds, beans, or legumes first, which greatly enhances digestion. Instead of merely avoiding these fabulous foods, give sprouting a try. Once sprouted, they are insanely good for you and your tired, pissed off tummy.

Soaking beans and seeds before you consume them helps to neutralize the enzyme inhibitors present in sproutable foods, such as grains and seeds. The process assists in the production of many beneficial enzymes, while simultaneously breaking down and neutralizing any phytic acid that may be lurking. Soaking and sprouting also helps to break down some otherwise semi-indigestible proteins into simpler, more easily absorbable components.[224] This is why it's important to soak dry beans overnight before you cook with them.

Grains, seeds, and beans sprout very easily; usually it only takes a few days. Some of my favorite items to sprout are chickpeas, lentils, and sunflower seeds.

How to Sprout

Step 1: Soak your fare overnight. Once you're ready to begin the process, drain the water and rinse them well. Throw away anything that looks mouldy, dark, broken, or generally different than the others. You want to look for uniformity.

Step 2: Keeping them damp, place them in a glass jar (I use Mason jars or old jam and pickle jars) and seal with a cheesecloth over the top, securing with an elastic. You don't want them sitting in visible water, you only want them damp. If they dry, just get them damp again.

Step 3: Keep the jar out of the sun, because otherwise they will leaf and/or dry out too fast. You only want them to sprout, which takes hours to a few days to accomplish. Natural sunlight is okay; just don't place the jar directly in the sun.

Step 4: Your eats are ready when the root is the length of the body. For example, if you are sprouting chickpeas, they are ready when the root is approximately one centimetre long.

Step 5: Store the sprouts in your refrigerator (in the jar) until you eat them all; they last about seven to ten days. My favorite things to do with sprouts are to throw them in salads, eat them on toast with hummus, on a sandwich or veggie burger, or just eat them plain. They are delish, and your tummy will be thankful.

Juicing

When I think or talk about juicing, I get super excited. If you are someone who truly wants to make a difference to your health, particularly digestive health, you'll need and want a juicer.

My first juicer came second-hand from my mother-in-law, and I intended to use it for a quick cleanse. I did that cleanse, and my love affair with juicing took flight. Making fresh juice every morning has become a ritualistic part of my morning routine. I get up, and I make juice. It makes me feel hydrated after a long night with little fluids, it keeps me regular, and it provides me with energy that I did not previously know existed. I've included my five favorite juice recipes in this chapter, including a beginner juice, a breakfast juice, an intermediate juice, my very favorite green juice, and an anti-inflammatory juice. I make the green juice every single morning, and if I feel like I need more energy, or if I think I might be getting sick (which rarely happens anymore), I juice more throughout the day. You can also partake in juice cleanses by juicing and drinking a lot of herbal tea all day long. You will also want to incorporate some miso soup into your cleanse days, for the purpose of replenishing important, depleted electrolytes. Don't substitute the soup for a sport drink; they are high in sugar and artificial yucky stuff. (Some are neon colored; that would be your first clue!) If the idea of miso soup is not turning your crank, then substitute in sixteen ounces of coconut water throughout the day, instead.

Cleaning house: I recommend just one or two days of cleansing, unless you feel strongly that you could use a few extra days of this due to constipation. See a naturopath for more instruction on juice cleanses that last longer than the weekend.

I own a Breville Juice Fountain Compact. It is a centrifugal juicer, which means that is has a very fast grater to shred the produce and then separate the juice from the pulp. Centrifugal juicers are cheaper than the alternatives, which are masticating and twin-gear juicers. These ones are more expensive, because they do a better job of getting all of the juice out of your produce. However, they are slower, cost more, and generally take up more space on your counter. All of the Breville juicers are great, and the one I own was purchased for about $125.00. When you are shopping for a juicer, consider the following:

- Will it be easy to clean? (Is it easy to take apart?)
- Is it quiet(ish)?
- What is the warranty? Make sure it's at least a year.
- How high is the spout, and is the spout dripless? You'll want it high enough to fill a ten to fourteen ounce glass.
- How big is the chute? The less you have to prep your produce, the better. My juicer's chute can fit a small apple, a whole cucumber, etc. I don't want to cut food up if I don't have to.

Juicing Tips

- Juice more when you feel that you might be coming down with a bug, or if you are low in energy.
- Use organic produce for juicing, because you will be absorbing everything that juice has to offer, and you want high levels of prime nutrients. It's a good reason to invest in organic produce, even if it's just for juicing.

- Juice items with the least water content first, ending with the items with the most water content. This is in order to flush out anything left in the juicer. For example: roots first, (like ginger, carrots, and beets), celery, lettuce, and hard fruit next, then apples, pears, etc. Cucumbers are always last.
- Juice on an empty stomach for prime nutrient absorption. (First thing in the morning is best.)
- Clean your juicer right after using it, so that the produce doesn't dry and cake onto the machine and the blade. It's just easier.
- Keep your juicer on the counter to remind you to use it daily. My husband hates anything on the counter, but I stand my ground with my juicer! And my mixer. And my herbs . . .

The following recipes make twelve to eighteen ounces of glorious juice. Juice in the given order:

Beginner Juice: One tiny piece of ginger, three large apples, and three large pears.

Breakfast Juice: Small piece of ginger, four large carrots, and two large grapefruits.

Intermediate Juice: Piece of ginger the size of your thumb, one small beet, four carrots, and two large apples. (I like one square inch of ginger, but that might be too spicy for you. Throw some celery in there if you want.)

Green Juice: Three romaine lettuce or chard leaves, two celery stalks with leaves, two pears or apples, and one large cucumber. Throw in a carrot or a few mint or basil leaves if you feel like getting creative. I make this juice every morning without fail. It makes me feel hydrated, and starts my day off with great nutrients.

Anti-Inflammatory Juice: Four to six fennel stalks with fronds, two celery stalks, two red apples, and one cucumber. This juice is great for days you are feeling less than fabulous: especially if you are experiencing bloating, or even a flare-up. The fennel is very anti-inflammatory, and the whole drink is fabulous for rehydration and bowel stimulation. Items such as mint and ginger are great in recovery juices, too.

Wheatgrass is one superfood that I love to grow. It is known for its alkalizing and anti-inflammatory effects on the body, as well as it being an antioxidant, opening up blood vessels, enriching the blood supply and helping digestive function. I purchase wheatgrass seeds at the health food store, and they take about six or seven days to get around four inches tall. Once they are about a week to a week and a half old, I cut them at their base and juice them in a vegetable blend. I have a trick for juicing them, because I don't own a masticating juicer. (If you ever order a wheatgrass shot at a juice bar, they use a masticating juicer.) I open up a lettuce or chard leaf, place my grass down the middle, put a carrot on top, roll the leaf up tight, and juice it like that. It works! Wheatgrass is incredibly good for you, and super fun to grow from seed. If you have kids, they will love to see how fast it happens. Get them involved and share good health by setting a good example. I love to visit juice bars and order a wheatgrass shot. Usually you will also be given a chaser for it, like pineapple juice. It wakes me up much better (and faster) than coffee ever could. Trade your java for juice, and attain a whole new level of perkiness!

When you are done running the produce through your juicer, go back and scoop up the fiber and pulp that has been discarded and run it through again. It's a great way to use up every last bit, and get the most juice for your buck. The left over pulp can either be mixed into soups and stews, or easily be added to your compost heap if you have one. It's an organic vegetable garden's aphrodisiac!

Helpful Kitchen Equipment

When you make the decision to stop eating yucky food, and start eating real food that makes you feel better, you might find that you want to invest in some new kitchen tools. If you are going to begin cooking with new and sometimes quite foreign foods, having the right tools for the job cuts down on any initial frustration you may have. Within the first year of my diet change, I bought a juicer, a food processor, a bamboo sushi mat, and a rice cooker. While keeping in mind that you don't need any of these items to get healthy, this is my list of what I personally consider kitchen must-haves for those who want to get cooking, and want to have fun while doing it:

1. Food chopper. This handy device can chop things like onions in seconds, and doesn't process them to the point of mush. All my friends have heard me say that I will never cut an onion with a knife again. My crying days are over—my children are no longer confused when I cook dinner.

2. Food processor. Great for soups, anything with alot of veggies in it like chili, salsa, guacamole, hummus, and more. I own both a manual one for small tasks, and a larger one for big jobs.

3. Juicer. I use this every day, and can't imagine life without it. The juice I make every morning is what keeps me in routine, hydrated, grounded, and regular.

4. Mixer. I use this on a weekly basis. I know this sounds spoiled, but I don't want to mix dough with a spoon anymore. I'm a lazy cook, and having help like this actually motivates me to hang out in the kitchen, instead of a restaurant.

5. A great knife. Actually, a few great knives. Sharp ones. My favorite kind of knife for general, everyday cutting is a santoku knife.

6. Stainless steel pots and pans. These are a must. Teflon ones are bad for you, because they contain carcinogen material that can enter the food being cooked with it. Remember, any little bit of help you can give your body, do it. Cast-iron is also a great way to go.

7. Blender. Very useful for making smoothies, which my entire family enjoys on a daily basis. It's a great way to fit in a quick, nutritious snack.

8. Bamboo sushi mat. You will get a lot of use from this. One of our favorite things to bring to our friends' houses and serve at our own home now is homemade vegetable rolls. They are super fun, and taste amazing.

9. Rice cooker. This device makes meal planning a cinch. I use it to make rice, millet, couscous, quinoa, and other whole grains.

10. Crock pot. A crock pot is fabulous to have, especially in the winter months. Homemade soups, stews, chili, and other plant-based dinners can be made while you are at work. Also, your house smells amazing all afternoon long!

11. Salad spinner. I use this handy tool every single day to quickly dry lettuce and kale. It saves me tons of time, and I can't imagine not having it now.

Stress and Nutrition

The effects of stress are dangerously underrated by most of us. Stress can be both good and bad, but more often than not, stress causes us considerable concern, and often on a daily basis. So, what exactly is stress? Stress is strain on the body and/or mind that causes our adrenal glands to release cortisol into our bloodstreams. Once used almost solely as a "fight or flight" response, this cortisol release happens far too often in our western life. Stressors no longer include predatory animals or the challenge of scavenging for food. Now our bodies perceive stress to be anything from mild environmental pollutants to the spicy food from that amazing Thai restaurant down the street. Your digestive system is incredibly sensitive to stress, and reflects that sensitivity by shutting itself down on a dime, or quickly powering up unnecessarily.

Stress is a bitch. It screws with our perception of things, our immune systems, our sleep, and our digestive performance. There are many stressors in our lives, and some people get more stressed out than others. (This is where I sheepishly raise my hand.) When I was deep into my IBS years, any type of stress would set off an attack, good or bad. Even things like getting in a good, hard, abdominal work-out would prompt swift guttural protests. If you can avoid stress, or try to cut it back, your body will be forever grateful.

It's also important to note that there are mixed views on whether or not IBS is caused by stress. My very first episode of IBS that I can remember coincided with a bad relationship. While I don't know for sure if my condition was sparked by the stress I went through during those few months, I do know that stress seemed to make my symptoms worse when coupled with an impending or existing flare-up. My personal opinion is that stress *does* contribute to IBS, or at least it did for me. I think that when your digestive system is clogged and inefficient, stress can contribute to the process of digestion (or lack thereof), in some way or another, whether it be significant or minimal.

Nutritional stress is defined by Brendan Brazier in his book *The Thrive Diet*, as "a stress created by food because of its unhealthy properties."[225] In layman's terms, the food you eat can either help you or stress your body out. We need all the nutrients we can get, for as little digestive work it takes. By eating strong, plant-based food, such as raw or slightly steamed vegetables, minimal stress is placed on your body, and you get the most bang for your buck in terms of energy output. When you eat something highly processed, your body works hard to digest it, and that creates additional stress. Ditto for meat and dairy.

Once you eliminate animal products from your diet and introduce whole, unprocessed foods, your body will respond positively and almost instantaneously, and you'll realize that you're completely capable of healing that troublesome tummy. With knowledge comes power, and honey, you'll want to be president of the Healthy Colon Club!

Other means of reducing stress, primarily by getting more sleep and increasing the quality of your exercise, will be next on your to-do list. Learning how to reduce stress will help you move your bowels better, curtail intestinal flare-ups, and ease stomach pain when you are in the middle of an episode.

Sleep, Baby, Sleep!

One excellent way to combat stress is to get enough sleep. I know research typically states that we should be getting seven to eight hours of beauty sleep per night, but I would like to argue that I need nine or ten! My husband often jokes that I'm neither a morning, nor a night person. Sleep is good, my friend. Get lots. How do we make sure our zzzz's are quality? Eat good, clean food. Also, try not to eat anything after dinner, so that when you go to bed, you are not still digesting it. Go to bed early, no later than ten o'clock if you can. Your body needs to repair and restore at night, and if it's concerned with digestion, that won't happen. Try having a bath with some epsom salts, or sip some warm chamomile tea. Maybe stretch a bit first, or meditate for five minutes. Sleep in the dark, and make sure your room is cool. It's also a good idea to try and go to bed at the same time every night, and wake at the same time every morning. This puts your body on a sleep cycle that it will recognize, and hopefully lead to more restful nights. Lack of sleep and constant exposure to stressors are correlated to weight gain, too, so getting enough consistent sleep could restoratively help you lose a few extra pounds that may be lingering for that very reason.

Another good way to make sure you stay stress-free is to exercise on a regular basis. Exercising is a fabulous stress reliever, and relieving stress will help you sleep better, too. See? It's a crazy cycle! Exercising does not have to be heavy weight lifting, by the way. Exercise should elevate your heart rate, while rhythmically stretch and massage your organs. Walking is a great way to accomplish this, and it also helps to stimulate your bowels. One of my favorite exercises is yoga. I leave a yoga class feeling light, optimistic, relaxed, and regenerated. Remember that treating your body well does not stop at food. Be nice to it in every way you know how.

Breathe . . .

The next suggestion that I have for you involves such a basic movement, yet is entirely necessary in order to detoxify, regenerate, and even live. Breathing is something that is often much overlooked and almost always under-practiced. The art of breathing in order to relax goes back to such ancient practices as yoga. Do you ever just sit in a quiet place and breathe? I often forget that doing such a thing is an option, but when I remember, I try and practice it on the spot. Deep breathing provides oxygen to our entire body and provides aid in clearing the mind, while achieving the sought-after state of parasympathetic nervous system dominance, "which is responsible for all healing, proper digestion, hormone balance, and a feeling of general well-being."[226] Remember the rule of tens: inhale deeply for a count of ten, exhale slowly for a count of ten, and then repeat it ten times. This is extremely relaxing and stress reducing. Remembering to do this routinely at least twice a day will be very helpful in delivering your blood cells the extra oxygen that they need. This breathing exercise can also be incredibly helpful in reducing pain that may have already settled in for a visit. Breathe deep, and send that unwanted visitor on a sabbatical!

> Stress buster: Stress is known to deplete mineral sources, which are important to proper digestive function. Relieving your stress will not only aid you psychologically, but also physically.

You Need to Relax (Om . . .)

It seems like a funny thing to say, but most of us don't know how to slow down and chill out anymore. North America is known throughout the world as a busy, crazy, hectic place to live and work. (Except for a few glorious regions in Mexico. . . .) We want to do everything, right now, really well, and in record time. Well, as the offspring of a classic type-A father, I can tell you that I used to be a pretty wound-up kinda girl. While there is huge correlation between eating more meat, more crap and less nutrients and being sicker than ever before, I also think that we could correlate the massive influx in sickness with our desire to be super-humans. Digestive disease is something that can definitely be brought on by rushed eating, too much eating, not eating, and stress eating. Maybe we need to take the time to enjoy eating our food, appreciate our environment, listen to some music, and bask in the nature that surrounds us every single day.

Our world begins to align itself when we chill. We chew our food more slowly, we take longer to eat, and we make better food choices. We start to notice little bodily signals that we never took the time to pay attention to before. We breathe more deeply and think more clearly. Relaxing is important for many reasons, and it will certainly help you digest your food better.

Here's the bottom line: Find a way to reduce stress and help yourself relax. The implementation of the methods given, along with the right foods, will help your digestive system recover.

If You Flare

Even though I very rarely get flare-ups anymore, I now know what to do in order to quickly reduce inflammation and absolve any pain. When you feel an episode coming (sometimes you know it's going to happen for hours before you are in real trouble, and sometimes you only get a one-minute warning), the following things are recommended that you do immediately:

- Stop eating! Do not eat if you feel an impending flare-up. Food at this point will just amount to added stress to your digestive system that is clearly already fighting with you. Instead, start sipping warm herbal tea, preferably fennel, peppermint, ginger, or chamomile. These herbs will help with inflammation and stomach upset.

- Lay flat on your back, with a warm towel or heating pad on your lower abdomen for about ten minutes. Once you remove it, gently massage your stomach clockwise; in the direction that food must travel through the colon. Yoga is also helpful; there are many positions that help massage the organs that are related to the digestive system.

- Aromatherapy oils help too. Anise and peppermint combinations are the best. You can lie down and apply the oil straight to your lower abdomen, while massaging it. Or, apply the oil to your wrists, and then lay an arm gently over your face and breathe it in, also while lying down. Deep, rhythmic breathing helps supply oxygen to your body, including your digestive system. It's extremely beneficial.

- If an episode begins while you are eating or shortly thereafter, it might be a good idea to get up and go for a walk. This helps to stimulate your bowel to work through what might be accumulated there. The fresh air and exercise also aids to achieve higher levels of oxygen intake.

- Sometimes it helps to take a very warm bath. You can also add the aromatherapy oils to it. The warms water helps to alleviate pain, and is also bowel stimulating.

- After you feel the flare-up begin to pass, be very aware of what you are eating. Continue with herbal tea and lots of tepid warm water. If you have IBS-D, you can try eating select foods that will slow your bowel down, such as sprouted grain breads, brown rice, bananas, and applesauce. (The BRAT diet.) Do not drink any caffeine or alcohol; your tummy needs to heal.

Natural Supplements

Consider holistic supplements that can help soothe your irritated gut right away:

- Peppermint Oil: aids in nausea, cramping, and gas.
- Papaya Enzymes: natural digestive enzymes that work very quickly.
- Aloe Vera Capsules: contributes to improved bowel mobility, reduced inflammation and pain, and possesses detoxification properties.
- Oil of Oregano: Reduces nausea and indigestion, strengthens the immune system, possesses antibacterial properties, and is anti-parasitic, antifungal, and antiviral.

Tips for Creating Bowel Movements Naturally (Sans Laxatives)

- Drink lots of room-temperature water. Water will help lubricate every part of the digestive system. Making sure that the water isn't cold is very helpful, because cold water shocks you internally, which is operating at a very warm 98.6 degrees Fahrenheit. Warm water works better, because then the body isn't offended by cold temperatures. (Simply heat cold water by warming in a pot or a kettle, but not by using hot water directly from the tap, as it can be contaminated with heavy metals from your hot water tank.) Water is essential in the process of cleanly moving along food matter in your small intestine, and also in being able to lubricate your colon in order to pass pain-free stools. Get used to drinking about eight glasses a day, and this action alone will help constipation considerably.
- Drink warm herbal teas, especially in the morning and on an empty stomach. Warm tea first thing upon waking will stimulate your bowels, and prompt swift movement. Warm lemon water is great, also, especially because lemon has an alkalizing effect. A pinch of cayenne pepper will further stimulate a bowel movement.

- Exercise. Move your body just by going for a walk. The action of walking massages your digestive parts, such as your stomach, intestines, and your colon.

- Eating fruit or drinking fresh juice. Fruit is full of enzymes that promote bowel function, and they act quickly. (Most fruit is fully digested and ready to be expelled within an hour or two.) Take care to juice your own fruits and veggies in order to take advantage of living enzymes. Store-bought juice doesn't possess the same nutritional benefits.

- Make sure you are getting enough *good* fats. Fat helps to lubricate the digestive process and bring about bowel movements more easily. Remember that there is quite a significant difference between good and bad fats. Foods like avocados, olives, and sweet potatoes can help move stool more easily. Bad fats, such as trans or saturated fats will further aggravate the problem.

- Raw veggies, beans, and whole grains should always leave you very regular and cleaned up. If you are eating a whole food, plant-based diet such as the one promoted in this book, you should not ever have trouble with bowel movements. If you genuinely are following this plan and still have concerns, you should talk to your doctor about arranging a colonoscopy or another medical procedure to see if there could be another cause for your symptoms that might be out of your realm of control.

Question: What was your favorite part of this chapter? What got you most excited? I recommend that you begin with what interests you most, and move on from there. Don't feel like you have to drop everything and incorporate all of this tomorrow, because that by itself would be a cause for stress! Go at your own pace; it took me two years. In fact, I'm still getting there. What will you change, add, or try first?

Highlight: Panchakarma and Its Role in Digestion

Panchakarma is something that I originally heard of during a yoga class. It immediately struck a chord with me, and I love its message and meaning; one of immense importance.

Essentially, Panchakarma is the Ayurvedic science of detoxification and rejuvenation. Ayurveda means "the knowledge of life." It is the traditional healing science in India, which is well known to be the birthplace of yoga. Ayurveda views chronic disease as the result of living life out of harmony, and out of balance with our environment, ourselves, and ultimately the universe. Ayurvedic methods of re-establishing this balance include diet, herbs, meditation, colonic therapy, aromatherapy, yoga, and Panchakarma.[227]

Panchakarma is the traditional route of detoxification for the cluttered mind and body. While there are many toxins in everyone's modern-day environments, Panchakarma is aimed at removing one specific offender: ama. Ama is an especially harmful toxin that in formed within our bodies, and is believed to be the product of improper digestion. It is supposedly the most damaging force in our body, and it contributes to chronic digestive disease. Panchakarma is what is used in Ayurveda to remove ama and restore our natural balance within our bodies.[228]

The process of Panchakarma is fairly specific, but in short terms, the patient goes through a detoxification process that allows the ama to exit the body through the digestive tract, and thus allows for balance and tranquility within the body to occur. This is achieved through special foods (all vegan), herbs, massage, steam, meditation, and sinus irradiation achieved by means of a neti pot.

I think Panchakarma resonates with me because it becomes so clear that proper digestion is paramount to living disease-free. We just don't pay enough attention to that part of ourselves, and that's too bad. Good digestion is so good for us, and bad digestion is so, so bad for us. Also, I think that it's important to note that the topic of digestive importance is not a new thing. Since Panchakarma has been practiced in some parts of the world for thousands of years, obviously good digestion was revered back then, too.

Namaste . . .

Chapter 11

Food Rules

"Eat food. Not too much. Mostly plants."[229]

—Michael Pollan, *In Defense of Food*

Here are the top five worst foods for digestive health, and the top five best. None of these should come as a surprise by now, but sometimes repetition can help to hit the lesson home. Y'know?

Top Five Worst Foods for Digestion:

1. Fried anything. Frying food at crazy high temperatures changes the properties of that food. You damage anything nutritious and instead, add some trans-fats and carcinogens to your plate. Hungry?

2. Red meat. Although you know by now that I advocate for the cessation of meat-eating when it comes to healthy digestion for a huge variety of reasons, red meat takes the cake here. It is simply too heavy and acidic to be digested properly. Period. We were not designed to consume it, and it will definitely make digestion so much harder if you try. If you're still not sure about this, I have a challenge for you.

Go strictly vegetarian for two weeks. On day fifteen, eat a six ounce steak. You'll wish you hadn't, but at least you'll know for sure.

3. Dairy. Again, this is a food that we are not supposed to consume. It is too high in fat, and we are intolerant to its proteins and sugars. It causes gas, bloating, and nausea. Not a good idea, amigos.

4. Alcohol. Once you stop crying for your loss just like I did, drink this up: alcohol slows digestion and overworks our liver and pancreas. There is nothing healthy about it. However, if you immensely enjoy a glass of red wine from time to time, then do it. The stress relief obtained by having a relaxing glass of wine a couple of times a week is worth it for me, and might be worth it for you too. Just don't go crazy. One glass—just make it a good one!

5. Anything genetically modified. For reasons outlined in the chapter seven, genetically modified food is dangerous and is quite possibly a primary contributor of crazy gut distress. Avoid these foods completely, and buy organic to be sure.

Top Five Best Foods for Digestion:

1. Raw vegetables and fruit. Eating these foods in their whole, raw form will provide your body with all the necessary antioxidants, enzymes, soluble fiber, and other nutrients it could ever ask for. These foods are a complete must for improved digestion.

2. Whole grains. Whole grains, such as brown rice, barley, quinoa, millet, buckwheat, and oats, are a huge source of insoluble fiber, meaning that they help sweep your digestive tract clean of sticky, inflammation-causing debris. They are essential for maintaining a clean, healthy colon. It is not the same if you consume the processed versions, such as breads and pastas. Eat the whole grain.

3. Healthy fats. Foods high in healthy fats, such as coconut, avocados, raw nuts, and olives are definitely crucial to digestive health. Don't cut these because of their caloric content – they possess a wealth of nutrition that is good for the heart, as well as lubrication for your digestive tract. Very important.

4. Sprouts. Teeming with live enzymes, these wee wonders are incredibly good for intestinal health. There are several different varieties available, or make your own.

5. Water. Seems obvious, doesn't it? Well, it can't be overlooked. Let's face it: without proper hydration, we would not be able to function, and we would cease to live. We absolutely require water for a number of things, including proper digestion. One of the most common digestive complaints is constipation, and just by doubling your daily water intake, you can easily begin to rid yourself of that unpleasant situation. (As well as ward off any emerging BFFs . . .)

Essential Nutrients

"Many studies have shown that vegetarians
seem to have a lower risk of obesity, coronary
heart disease (which causes heart attack),
high blood pressure, diabetes mellitus and
some forms of cancer."[230]

—The American Heart and
Stroke Association

There are many misconceptions about what a plant-based diet can provide in terms of essential nutrients that are deemed necessary in order to be healthy. The following nutritional intake items (protein, carbohydrates, fat, micronutrients, iron, vitamin B12, and fiber), seem to be of particular concern to people when approached with the concept of a vegetarian diet (particularly a vegan one). In response to this, let me address these items one at a time:

Macronutrients

Protein

Protein is required by the body for proper growth, maintenance and repair of all your body's cellular components. It is needed for the creation of antibodies, which are the key to fighting against infection and illness. It keeps our nails strong, our bones healthy, our hair shiny, and our skin young and resilient. Protein is also a major contributor to all muscles, tissues and organs, and plays an invaluable role in regards to metabolism, digestion and nutrient transportation via oxygen within the circulatory system.

On a global scale, plant-based protein sources make up about 60% of human protein intake. In the United States and Canada, approximately 70% of our protein comes from animal sources.[231]

Proteins are made up of long chains of amino acids. There are twenty-two different types of amino acids and the body needs all of them to function properly. There are divided into two groups: essential and non-essential. The body cannot produce essential amino acids itself, and therefore they must be sourced from the food that we eat. Contrary to this, non-essential amino acids can be manufactured by the body and do not have to be derived from food.[232]

There are some foods that contain all of the essential amino acids required to form the new proteins together with the non-essential amino acids. These foods are called "complete" proteins and are strongly associated with animal products. They are found in meat, fish, shellfish, poultry and dairy products. The proteins that are termed "incomplete" proteins are usually lacking in one or more of the essential amino acids. They are generally found in plant sources, like fruits, vegetables, beans, grains and nuts. However, by combining two or more of the incomplete proteins, a complete supply of essential amino acids becomes available. For example, brown rice and beans will form a complete protein and give the body all the essential amino acids.

Since you are on a path to not eating animal products anymore in an effort to make peace with your digestive system (wave that white flag!), products such as tofu and quinoa are both excellent sources of readily available complete proteins.

It is important to understand that you do not need to create complete proteins in the same meal. Your body will store nutrients and pair them when they are made available.[233] See? Easier than you thought, right? It's also worth acknowledging that we are often told that we need way more protein than we actually do—as in, three or four times as much. In fact, protein deficiency is highly unheard of in developed countries. In contrast to the popular fear of not ingesting enough protein, too *much* protein can actually hurt us, so feel confident knowing that your protein intake, while adopting a plant-based diet, will be just fine.[234]

Myth: you won't get enough protein if you don't eat meat. Fact: if you are eating a plant-based diet, with a lot of variety and attention to good foods, you are definitely getting enough protein.

Percentage of Calories from Protein (Value Per 100 Grams Edible Portion)

From the U.S. Department of Agriculture's National Nutrient Database for Standard Reference, 2009:

Fruits

Apple 2%	Cantaloupe 10%
Banana 5%	Grapefruit 8%
Grapes 4%	Pineapple 4%
Honeydew melon 6%	Strawberry 8%
Orange 8%	Tangerine 6%
Papaya 6%	Tomato 19%
Peach 9%	Watermelon 8%
Pear 3%	

Grains

Barley 14%

Brown rice 8%

Buckwheat 15%

Millet 12%

Oatmeal 17%

Rye 18%

Wheat germ 26%

Wheat (hard red) 15%

Wild rice 16%

Legumes, Raw

Garbanzo beans 21%

Kidney beans 58%

Lentils 34%

Lima beans 24%

Navy beans 37%

Soybeans 35%

Split peas 29%

Nuts and Seeds

Almonds 15%

Cashews 13%

Filberts 9%

Peanuts 18%

Pumpkin seeds 18%

Sesame seeds 12%

Sunflower seeds 16%

Walnuts (black) 15%

Vegetables, Raw

Artichokes 28%

Beets 15%

Broccoli 33%

Brussels sprouts 31%

Cabbage 24%

Cauliflower 32%

Cucumbers 17%

Eggplant 17%

Green peas 27%

Green pepper 17%

Kale 26%

Lettuce 36%

Mushrooms 56%

Mustard greens 41%

Onions 9%

Potatoes 18%

Spinach 50%

Turnip greens 20%

Watercress 84%

Yams 5%

Zucchini 30% [235]

Carbohydrates

Oh Atkins, how you've messed with our heads. Nowadays, if you ask someone how they plan on shedding a few pounds, most people would reply by cutting back on carbs. Being overweight, or even obese, has been blamed on carbohydrates for far too long. We need to start educating ourselves properly and becoming accountable for our own food choices.

Here's the truth: we need carbohydrates in order to live. Without them, we would die. Period. I'm not talking about jelly doughnuts or pasta primavera; I'm talking about good ole' whole grains and fresh fruit. You know—the food that provides us with long-lasting energy and bulk for our stool. Carbohydrates provide us with our energy and fiber, and all carbohydrate sources originate from plants.

There are two types of carbohydrates: simple and complex. Simple carbohydrates, when eaten, absorb quickly throughout your blood stream, and cause your pancreas to panic. When it freaks out, it creates a lot of insulin, which is an attempt to bring your glucose levels back to normal. The sugar high comes fast and hard, but once our glucose levels are straightened out by our stressed-out pancreas, we crash. We store the metabolised sugar, and it turns to fat. In short, we go up, we go down, our body wears itself out, and then we put on weight. Simple carbohydrates include anything with refined added sugars, white breads and pastas, confectionaries, candy, alcohol, etc. These foods will screw with you.

In his book *In Defense of Food*, Michael Pollan writes, "Deficiency diseases are much easier to trace and treat . . . than chronic diseases, and it turns out that the practice of refining carbohydrates is implicated in several of these chronic diseases as well-diabetes, heart disease, and certain cancers."[236] In other words, an overabundance of simple sugars can cause health issues so great that they are totally connected to three of the worst chronic diseases that we see far too often in the west.

> Disappearing Act: Western diseases virtually cease to exist with the introduction of a whole food, plant-based diet, in large part because if you are interested in keeping such a healthy diet, you aren't eating the crap that is associated with a more carnivorous one.

The reaction to complex carbohydrates is much different. When consumed, they slowly get dispersed throughout our blood stream. This gives us smaller, but steadier amounts of energy to work with. Our pancreas creates less insulin because it does not panic, and that way there is no crash. We metabolize the sugar, and we don't need to store it. We don't gain weight. Complex carbohydrates include all sprouted whole grains, and all fruit and vegetables, especially sweeter ones, such as beets, carrots and yams. Eat these; they are not the enemy. The two types of carbohydrates are not created equal. Complex is good, and simple is bad.

Myth: you'll consume far too many carbohydrates on a plant-based diet. Fact: while carbohydrates do become much more of a focus on this plan, you will be way more educated on what types of carbohydrates are necessary (complex), and which ones are trouble makers (simple). Carbohydrates are completely necessary to pair with other nutritious foods, such as beans and vegetables, in order to create complete proteins. They are also needed for their insoluble fiber to aid in proper elimination.

Finally, we can call carbs our friend. Go on, dance in the street! Shout it to the rooftops!

Fat

Ah, the lubricant of life! This nutrient is really an important one that is very often overlooked or underestimated because of today's misconceptions of it. Fat is a key component to our diet; you just have to be sure that you are eating the right kind, and of course, the right amount.

There are two different categories of fats: good fats, which are composed of essential fatty acids, such as omega 3, 6, and 9, and bad fats, which include saturated fats and trans-fatty acids. The good fats are what keep our skin glowing, contribute to bowel regularity, and make our hair shiny. Bad fats contribute to clogged arteries, heart disease, and raised cholesterol levels.

Good fats are in foods such as olives, avocados, raw seeds, raw nuts, and coconut. These fats play a vital role in brain function. The term "essential fatty acids" literally means that these fats are essential. We need them. The less refined a fat, the better it is for you.

The trick with fats is to eat a relatively low-fat diet, but that doesn't mean you should buy products that are advertised as being low in fat, or no-fat. These products are highly processed and in order to make the product edible, a ton of sugar is injected into the product to make up for the fat that was taken out. This goes back to the whole food being better than the sum of its parts. Eat foods that contain good fats in moderation, and eat them in their whole form. Omega 3 and 6 fatty acids should be consumed in a 1:1 ratio, ideally.[237] This ratio is achieved easily and naturally when you're consuming a healthy, varied diet.

Bad fats are mostly found in animal meat and processed foods; especially fast food. The food that is the very highest in bad or saturated fats is ground beef. High levels of saturated fats are also found in dairy and most baked goods. To avoid illness and efficiently rebuild intestinal health, it's important to totally avoid hydrogenated oils, such as margarines and shortenings, and other oils that are heated above 320 degrees Fahrenheit, which includes all fried foods.

Myth: vegetarians are skinny and unhealthy, due to consuming low amounts of fat. Fact: vegetarians do consume way less saturated fats (because that type of fat is mostly found in animal products), but it's very easy to make sure you get enough good fat in the form of avocados, olives, nuts, etc. You can be as healthy as you want to be.

Micronutrients

Vitamins and Minerals

Vitamins are abundantly present in whole grains, fruits, vegetables, beans, and nuts. The vitamins originally present in animal products debatably cease to exist after pasteurization of dairy, and high-heat cooking of meat. The very best ways to make certain that you obtain your vitamins is through consumption of plant products.

Vitamins are essential to our lives and our health, and we need to obtain them through our food. They are incredibly important in the aiding of digestive unease, and assisting to heal digestive upset. Taking vitamin supplements are not the same as ingesting your vitamins through whole foods, because whole foods have the exact right ratio of vitamins and also contain other substances that help their absorption.

A comprehensive list of vitamins that are associated with digestion is as follows: A (retinol), B (carotene), B1 (Thiamin), B2 (Riboflavin), B3 (Pyridoxine), B6 (Pantothenic Acid), B12 (Cobalamin), Biotin, Folic Acid, C Complex, D (cholecalciferol), and E (tocopherols).[238] All of these vitamins have functions that directly relate to intestinal health and repair.

Without minerals, we could not live. Minerals are extremely important to all bodily functions. Thankfully, Mother Nature has provided us with a plenitude of minerals, found in whole foods, such as fruits, vegetables, sea vegetables, whole grains, seeds, nuts, and beans. Eating a varied diet should ensure that you have all you need.

Low amounts of any mineral can contribute to poor digestive function. Because your digestive tract depends on proper mineral consumption in order to create digestive enzymes and repair itself, inadequate amounts of minerals could seriously inhibit your gut's ability to heal—something that an IBS sufferer (or any other digestive sufferer), cannot afford. Sugar and dairy products are known to deplete mineral storage, so high consumption of these foods is not recommended. As if you needed yet another reason to forgo the dairy!

The following are minerals that are essential for digestive tract repair: calcium, magnesium, sodium, potassium, iron, zinc, iodine, chromium, copper, manganese, selenium, and sulphur.[239] Because of the popular "am I getting enough iron?" concern with regards to a vegetarian diet, it will be addressed next:

Iron

> "Vegetarians do not have a higher incidence of iron deficiency than do meat eaters."[240]
>
> —The Vegetarian Resource Group

Iron is an essential mineral that is absolutely necessary for human life. Most of the iron in the body reside in the red blood cells that carry oxygen to each and every one of our cells. When not enough iron is present, cells become oxygen deprived, and so does your body in general. What results from this is anemia. The most easily recognizable symptoms of anemia are weakness and exhaustion. Iron deficiency is the number one nutritional disorder in the world, with an estimated up to 80% of people affected.[241] While vegetarians do have to be careful that they consume enough iron, so does the rest of the population. Red meat is high in iron, but depending on the age of the meat, how it's cooked, and the way the human body digests it, the amount of iron one actually obtains from it might be grossly overestimated. In fact, according to the National Cancer Institute, meat of any kind that is cooked at a high temperature, such as barbequed or grilled, actually becomes carcinogenic through the release of free radicals.[242] In other words, meat may contain iron, but its consumption is at the expense of it also possibly being cancer causing.

There are two types of iron you can obtain from food: heme and non-heme. There is conflicting information out there about whether heme or non-heme iron sources are best, in terms of actual absorption. Dietary sources of heme iron are liver and other organ meats, lean red meat, poultry, fish, and shellfish. This type of iron has long been touted as the best, because its absorption rate is faster than its sister. However, just as studies showing that plant protein is used less efficiently in our bodies than animal protein and that this is actually better for us in terms of less tumour growth and disease prevention,[243] non-heme iron's slower absorption rate is more favorable within the human body, since the body only uses what it needs, and this way, there is little chance of storing too much iron (which can happen). It's interesting how we are so programmed to think "bigger, better, faster," when in actuality, that way of thinking gets us into trouble more often than not.

Sources of non-heme iron include dried beans and peas, legumes, nuts and seeds, whole grains, dark molasses, and green leafy vegetables. There are some nutrients that help the body better absorb this kind of iron, and some that hinder its effectiveness. For example, vitamin C helps the absorption of non-heme iron, while caffeine, the tannins in tea, and calcium (including all dairy products) blocks its absorption. Also, too much iron can be constipating, which is something to be aware of if you experience digestive discomfort. Because of this, I don't recommend taking iron supplements unless suggested by a doctor to treat anemia. As long as you are following a clean, varied diet, your iron levels should not be a problem. (Tip: try cooking with a cast-iron frying pan!)

Myth: vegetarians don't get enough iron. Fact: plant-based eaters usually get more! Because individuals who embark on whole food, plant-based diets tend to be more health conscious in general than their counterparts, iron intake is often well taken care of. Personally, I flitted back and forth with anemia until I started eating plant-based. I am so much more educated now regarding what my body needs, that getting enough iron is a no-brainer for me. There is a ton of great, easily absorbable iron in green, leafy veggies, beans, and fortified grain products. Iron up!

When I give blood, the nurses usually tell me that my iron levels are fantastic, and are very surprised to learn I don't eat red meat. I didn't become a blood donor until I became a plant-based eater, because before that I was usually slightly anemic and was not permitted to donate with my previously low iron levels.

Vitamin B12

When I started my journey into Vegetable City, I was told that I should take a daily supplement to cover my B vitamins. Vitamin B12, in particular, is a water-soluble vitamin that is naturally found in some foods, added to others, is available as a supplement, and can be prescribed as a medication to those with very low levels. (People diagnosed with a B12 deficiency are often given B12 injections.) It is needed for red blood cell formation, brain function, and DNA synthesis.[244]

Vitamin B12 is naturally found in animal products, including fish, meat, poultry, eggs, milk, and milk products. It is generally not present in conventional plant foods, due to the obsession we currently have with over-cleaning our vegetables and poisoning our soil with pesticides and herbicides. If you grow your own organic vegetables, try not to scrub them clean. (This one will throw your kids for a loop!) Vitamin B12 is present in natural soil, and we need so little of it, that we can obtain it by eating lightly rinsed veggies. Fortified whole grain products are also a readily available source of vitamin B12, which is a good option for vegetarians. I take a B12 supplement every three days or so, and it is recommended that anyone embarking on a strict vegetarian diet do the same. (Note: just as beets turn your urine pink, B12 turns your pee bright yellow! Don't be alarmed.)

Myth: you won't get enough vitamin B12 on a plant-based diet. Fact: you will if you are aware that you need it.

Fiber

While many people don't consider fiber to be a micronutrient, I think it's worthy of some pedestal-action here. In his book *The China Study*, Dr. T. Colin Campbell writes, "high fiber intake was consistently associated with lower rates of cancers of the rectum and colon. High-fiber intakes were also associated with lower levels of blood cholesterol. Of course, high-fiber consumption reflected high plant-based food consumption; foods such as beans, leafy vegetables and whole grains are all high in fiber."[245]

There are two different types of fiber: soluble and insoluble. Soluble sources are oats, nuts, seeds, beans, most veggies and most fruits. Soluble fiber dissolves in water, making its nutrients readily available to the body, and slowly provides long-lasting energy. It is also important for lowering cholesterol and stabilizing blood sugar.

Insoluble fiber sources include dark, leafy greens, root vegetables, bran, corn, and fruit skins. They are not water soluble, which means they are pretty much indigestible. Sounds like a waste of food, but insoluble fiber is super important. It helps to absorb water, add bulk to waste, and help sweep it out of the colon. It's what gives your stool its shape and consistency, and contributes to your regularity and ease at which your bowel movements are performed. It helps prevent constipation, which can be extremely important to someone with diverticular disease, as well as IBS-C. Both types of fiber are incredibly necessary to consume. There is absolutely no fiber in animal meat or dairy. These foods throw your digestive tract off its preferred course, by either causing constipation (through consumption of meat) or an allergic, mucousy response (through consumption of dairy).

Fiber is our friend; don't take it for granted. Be aware of it, and try to eat a lot of it. That being said, make sure that if you are going to begin consciously eating more fiber, that you also drink more fluid.

Without the fluid, fiber can be constipating or create hard stool, which in turn might contribute to hemorrhoids. Just remember: fluid and fiber go together. Also, if you suffer from IBS-D or IBD, make certain that you and your doctor have a fiber plan. Fiber may be an initial problem for you if you are in the middle of a flare-up.

Myth: you'll be using the bathroom ten times a day if you try and eat more fiber. Fact: when you eat a varied, whole, plant-based diet, your body will probably detoxify at first and take a couple of weeks to adjust. After that, you will have regulated yourself perfectly, and your body will thank you by working exactly the way it's supposed to.

If you have digestive issues, whether accompanied by constipation or diarrhea, the right types of fiber will create balance and ground you. It will sweep you clean if you're constipated, and it will regulate you properly to ensure proper vitamin and mineral absorption if you are prone to diarrhea. Chronic constipation and diarrhea indicate intestinal inflammation and bacteria imbalance. A whole food, plant-based diet will correct these issues naturally, without the need for medication or intervention.

Enzyme pitch: Digestive enzymes are absolutely crucial to proper digestion. Their job is to properly break down food for absorption, without which, we would all be very malnourished and in a lot of digestive distress. Some of us are in this very serious predicament already. Here's the skinny on enzymes:

Enzymes are present in live food. That is, food that is either completely raw, or has been slightly heated to no more than 120 degrees Fahrenheit. You are not getting enough enzymes if you are not eating raw food, only eating processed and fully-cooked food, or if your body is chronically stressed.

You can increase your enzyme count in many different ways. You can eat more raw food. You can eat more sprouts and fermented vegetables, which are very high in enzymes. You can take enzyme supplements, such as digestive enzymes, prebiotics, and probiotics. If you have guttural issues such as IBS, you would highly benefit from these tiny lifesavers; I don't leave home without them. What are you waiting for? Go get your enzymes on!

Pantry Prerequisites

The following excerpt was taken from a joint report from the World Health Organization and the Food and Agriculture Organization of the United Nations:

"Households should select predominantly plant-based diets rich in a variety of vegetables and fruits, pulses or legumes, and minimally processed starchy staple foods. The evidence that such diets will prevent or delay a significant proportion of non-communicable chronic diseases is consistent."[246]

This section is my favorite. It is also the most important. Having your refrigerator, freezer, and pantry totally stocked with yummy, nutritious ingredients and snacks is essential. The secret to successfully obtaining all the nutrients you need and making the transition from an omnivorous, processed, "western" diet to a lighter, more healthful and whole, plant-based one is, in one word, variety. You need to make sure that you don't get bored, uninspired, or run out of good eats. Making sure that your kitchen is stocked for success is vital. I know every woman hates to hear this, but I'm afraid you're going to have to go shopping!

Raw plants, such as fresh veggies and fruit are obviously at the center of a plant-based diet—they're in the name! By keeping a wide variety of fruits and vegetables on hand, you will increase the variety of natural nutrients that each food possesses. Keep raw veggies cut and ready to go in the fridge, especially if you juice or blend. Try and purchase different kinds of apples and lettuce each week, or switch up what types of melon you have on hand. Variety means different foods, each with their own, unique blends of nutrients. I totally dare you to go to your local grocer and purchase five items from the produce section that you have never purchased before. It's kind of exhilarating! For the best quality produce, try to shop at local farmers markets or produce stands. Locally grown fruit and veggies have way more vitamins, because they are fresher. The longer an apple has to travel to get to you, the fewer amount of nutrients it will retain.

A giant variety of whole grains is essential; every grain that you purchase for your family should be whole. The nutritional difference between white bread and whole wheat bread is immense. For example, one slice of white bread has zero grams of protein, and zero grams of fiber. One piece of whole wheat bread has, on average, two grams of protein, and two grams of fiber. Better yet, one slice of spouted grain bread has up to ten grams of protein, and seven grams of fiber. Grains to become familiar with are brown rice, kamut, spelt, barley, oats, millet, buckwheat, and quinoa.

Beans are so incredibly important to a plant-based diet. These tiny powerhouses are absolutely teeming with protein, fiber, and other fantastic nutrients. My personal favorites are chickpeas, red kidney beans, lentils, and black beans. Although I do often use canned beans for a quick fix (no added salt, and sold in packaging containing no BPA), I also store dried lentils, kidney, and navy beans in my freezer. Dehydrated beans are super cheap, too. They fill you up, and lend great energy. There are tons of great dishes that center around the bountiful bean. Chili, black bean and corn quesadillas, and chickpea curries are always favorites at my house. Also, bean burritos, bean-filled pitas, and beans atop a salad are weekly ways that beans make it into my tummy. Soon, they will make their way into yours.

Sprouts. Yep—we are going there again. I know that most sprouts originate from a vegetable or bean, both of which I have already rallied for, but once these foods sprout, they become different. Because the seed or bean has been "sprouted," it contains active digestive enzymes that your body both needs and loves. Sprouts are so good for you, whether they are purchased pre-packaged, or you grow your own.

Tofu, seitan, and tempeh are excellent sources of a complete protein, because they are all soy products. They are also very versatile, but I urge you to experiment with different types and textures until you find a product that you love. Make sure you buy organic, because these foods are made from soy, and the majority of soy grown in the United States and Canada is genetically modified. Keep in mind that these foods are also processed, so maybe try and limit these products to a couple of times a week, max. The unrefined version of soy is the beans in their original pod. Called edamame (you might already be familiar with this, as many vegetarian-friendly restaurants offer this dish as an appetizer), they are delicious when steamed and sprinkled with sea salt.

Plant butters, such as peanut butter, almond butter (my fave), and cashew butter are key pantry staples. Tahini is good too. It's a sesame seed paste, and is also a great spread or base for a dip. (You can find these items in the health food aisle at your grocery store.) Each type has variances in their benefits, but all are fantastic plant-protein options for the meatless eater. Obviously, nuts themselves are also important to have on hand. Raw almonds are the best in terms of energy lent to the consumer with the least amount of fat content. Nuts are naturally chalk-full of good fat, protein, and essential fatty acids. They pack a large punch for their small size. Again, just be aware of the pesticide issue, and buy organic. Peanuts in particular are known to contain high quantities of toxins due to chemical sprays, so make sure you buy organic peanut butter, too. Store your raw nuts in the freezer to prolong freshness.

Seeds are so, so underrated. They are excellent snacks, and are full of great nutrients. Sunflower, pumpkin, flax and sesame seeds are definitely the most popular. You can eat them by themselves, or sprinkle them in baking, or on your salads or oatmeal. You can mix them in cereal, or even make your own trail mixes. Because many schools and workplaces are now "nut-free zones," a small container of seeds is a great replacement for the sadly banned, recently forbidden nut. I throw ground flax seed in everything. (Flaxseeds need to be ground to unleash their awesome nutrient-rich potential! We don't digest the seed easily if it's in its whole form.) Stir it in applesauce, blend it in smoothies, throw ¼ cup in spaghetti sauce, sprinkle it in baking. Flax, although relatively high in calories because it's a fantastic source of good fat, is also very high in both protein and fiber. It's too nutritionally important to not have on your refrigerator's shelf. Plus, you can sneak it into anything your kids (or partners) eat!

Frozen fruit is awesome to have on hand, because it makes smoothie creations easy and exciting. It's also a great way to use fruit that is too ripe to eat fresh. Freeze your softening strawberries, your bruised blueberries, and your brown bananas. Frozen fruit is also easy to blend and make your own homemade popsicles. Blend with coconut milk or water, organic soy yogurt, filtered water, or 100% juice (the only kind you should stock), and easy smoothies (and popsicles) can be made quickly and deliciously.

Healthy Habits: If you really want to get creative and tap into your inner health nut, blend your frozen fruit with some frozen broccoli, ½ an avocado, and a tablespoon of chia seeds in the blender. To sweeten your smoothies or popsicles, add a little bit of organic brown rice syrup or agave nectar. They are better products than plain old sugar, because they are much lower on the glycemic index, and provide a smoother sugar high, not a spike and subsequent crash. Stevia is another great sweetener, but be careful because it's about thirty times more sweet than cane sugar. Wowsers!

Cultured or fermented vegetables are virtually overlooked in our area of the world. Include them in your diet a couple of times a week in order to reap the enormous amount of benefits they offer. You can make them yourself, which is best, or you can purchase organic sauerkraut. Add them to sandwiches, veggie burgers, and salads. They are extremely high in digestive enzymes.

Sea vegetables such as kelp, dulse, arame and wakame, are excellent sources of iron, Vitamin C, iron, and digestive enzymes. I personally enjoy nori, which comes in a dried sheet, to help make things like wraps and vegetable rolls. These sheets are easy to prepare and store for a long time in your pantry. You can get them all at the health food store. Hint: please get them wet! You need to rehydrate the seaweed before you roll with it. Sounds silly to have to explain, but the first time I tried it, I totally dry-rolled and it was gross! Plus, I did it in front somebody who was fixing something in my kitchen for me. He thought I was super weird, I'm sure . . .

Meat alternatives are another fun food to have around in the first leg of your plant-based journey. Just be aware that they are highly processed, so they don't carry as much love as good ole' veggies and beans. Vegan ground round is an excellent alternative to ground beef, so you can use this for pasta, tacos, cabbage rolls, etc. Veggie hotdogs and burgers are also available, but I totally challenge you to make your own veggie burger patties out of mushrooms, nuts, beans, and other veggies. There are tons of great recipes out there. Speaking of convenience foods, I also personally love frozen, veggie pizzas. You can get them gluten-free and/or soy-free, even. Check these items out in the refrigerated sections of your local grocery store's health food aisle. Again, think of these foods as bridge foods. Start with these, and slowly wean yourself off by making your own food masterpieces. Processed food is simply not as good (in terms of taste and health) as homemade fare.

Tons and tons of easy-to-grab snacks are also great to have on hand. Consider organic, whole grain tortilla chips and salsa, plain popcorn, veggies and hummus, 100% fruit juice popsicles, soy yogurt cups, Clif Bars (high in protein; about twelve grams per bar; Chocolate Mint is my fave), Leslie Stow's Raincoast Crisps, fruit, apple slices and almond butter, edamame with sea salt, garlic-stuffed olives, homemade kale chips, etc. For the sweet tooth, my favorite guilty pleasure is organic, dark chocolate almonds or hard peppermint.

Natural sweeteners. Let's be honest: sometimes you need the sweet stuff. When you do, you don't want to bust yourself throwing back a tablespoon of refined sugar. (I've actually seen someone do that!) Better choices for toppings or baking are agave syrup, brown rice syrup, or stevia. These three sweeteners, as you have already seen, score lower on the glycemic index than their more refined friends, and therefore are a smoother ride than what other sweeteners can offer you. You want to avoid the spike and crash that inevitably accompanies refined sweeteners.

Condiments are absolutely essential to include in your dietary staples. If you are going to try new foods, they need to be accompanied by new flavors, sauces, and dips. Some of my favorites are Tamari (organic, gluten-free, super-tasty soya sauce), miso paste, miso bouillon cubes, wasabi, tahini dipping sauce, and curry paste. You will often find that these items are required in recipes that you will see in vegan and vegetarian recipe books. Another great new product to try is Daiya, a dairy, casein, lactose, gluten, and soy-free substitute for cheese. It makes it much easier to make such dishes as vegan lasagne. You can find all of these products in the health food aisle of your local grocery store. Embrace the new! Out with the yuck!

Supplements. Specifically, probiotics and vitamin B12, which are both highly beneficial to someone eating a plant-based diet. Probiotics are fabulous, because they provide friendly bacteria for your intestines, which help to keep the bad bacteria in check. Vitamin B12 has already been discussed a couple of times, so by now, it should be a no-brainer. If you feel that you may not be getting enough vitamins and minerals through your plant-based diet (maybe you're a picky eater?), then a good quality multivitamin should also help, in theory. That being said, if you are eating a varied plant-based diet, rich in raw veggies and whole grains, you probably won't need one. Again, always remember that a whole food is always better than the sum of its parts.

So, in conclusion of this section, here is your shopping list: fresh, organic, raw produce, whole grains, beans, tofu and tempeh (if you feel brave), organic nuts and nut butters, seeds, organic frozen fruit, healthy fats and cold-pressed oils, sea vegetables, picked vegetables, organic hemp, rice, almond, or soy milk, anything that looks interesting in the refrigerated section, low-fat, nutritionally high snacks, new cooking condiments, and the supplements that were just mentioned. Most of these items can be purchased from your local grocery store, but if your grocer doesn't stock them, they are sure to be found at your local health-food store. Keep these items on hand always. Yummy, quick, interesting food equals better success when you are modifying your diet.

Meal Ideas to Get You Started

Breakfast Ideas

- Fresh, organic juices (make your own)
- Good quality, whole-grain cereals with unsweetened, organic rice/hemp/soy/almond/coconut milk
- Homemade oatmeal topped with raisins, raw pumpkin seeds, and raw sunflower seeds
- Quinoa cooked with unsweetened almond milk instead of water, and banana slices
- Fresh, organic fruit, organic soy yogurt, and raw walnuts
- Smoothie with frozen fruit, avocado, flax oil, water (Add some organic soy yogurt if you want)

- Homemade muesli made with dry oats, coconut, thinly sliced organic apples, and almond milk
- Sprouted grain toast with almond or peanut butter (Silverhills Sprouted Bakery makes great sprouted bread)

Lunch/Dinner Ideas

- Black bean taco made on an organic corn tortilla, with homemade salsa, homemade coleslaw, lime, and cilantro
- Black bean quesadilla made with organic, soft corn tortillas, homemade salsa, cilantro, and lime
- Salad with seeds, nuts, avocados, chickpeas and/or roasted beets
- Lettuce wraps with portabella mushrooms, carrots, pea shoots, etc
- Portabella mushroom fajitas with organic, whole grain wraps, lettuce, homemade salsa, etc
- Homemade soups with veggie broth, beans, and veggies
- Homemade soup with pureed squash, etc
- Vegetarian sandwich made with sprouted grain bread, veggies, avocado, and hummus
- Amy's Organic Lentil Soup—you can buy this soup in bulk at Costco
- Vegetarian chili
- Vegetarian stew
- Open-faced veggie burgers (nut and bean mix) with pickled peppers, lettuce, and tomato on portabella mushroom "bun"
- Salad or vegetable rolls with wasabi
- Make your own pizza using whole wheat wraps or pita bread and soy cheese
- Whole wheat spaghetti with ground round and veggie tomato sauce
- Whole wheat pita stuffed with brown rice, beans, sprouts, cucumber, tomato, and tzaziki

Snack Ideas

- Sprouted grain bread with hummus and sprouts
- Raw nuts and seeds
- Kale chips
- Raw, organic veggies and dip
- Organic fruit and organic soy yogurt
- Clif Bars (some are totally vegan)
- Organic apple slices with almond, cashew or peanut butter
- Organic brown rice cake with tahini (sesame seed paste), drizzled with agave syrup
- Rice Works snacking chips
- Vegan seven-layer dip and good-quality tortilla chips (refried beans, guacamole, salsa, soy cheese, black olives, red and green peppers)
- Green olives stuffed with garlic

Sweet Cravings

- Dark, organic chocolate
- Dried fruit or fruit leathers (try making your own!)
- Organic soy or coconut ice cream
- Organic baked apples or pears, stuffed with cinnamon, oats, and a little agave syrup
- Organic apples, halved and stuffed with peanut butter and oats
- Chai tea sweetened with agave syrup or brown rice syrup
- 6 oz. glass of organic red wine (only if you know you don't have a sensitivity towards it).

Eating Consciously at a Restaurant, a Friend's Home, or On the Fly

Now that you have a good grasp of what kinds of foods you should be eating to soothe that exhausted, over-indulged, cranky tummy of yours, you certainly don't want to break your new routine by eating food that is not specially prepared by you. Here are some tips:

At a Restaurant

Don't feel as though you must only dine in vegan restaurants, but do try and stick to places that at least cater to vegetarians. Most restaurants do this, and at the very least you can order a salad. Also, don't be afraid to order something that is not listed on the menu. Think that chicken quesadilla looks good? Ask for a veggie version, and ask them to increase the veggie portion big-time, sans cheese if you don't plan on consuming dairy anymore. If the dish comes with fries, ask if you could upgrade to a salad. Most servers are used to special requests, and yours is not unreasonable as long as you're not ordering a clubhouse sandwich, no mayo, no meat, no wheat. What you're really asking for in that instance is a salad, so just order one.

At a Friend's Home

Find out what your friend is preparing to serve before you go, and ask if you can bring a veggie side dish. Then, at the very least, there is one item you can eat. It's also probably a good idea to let your friend know that you've decided to take on a whole food, plant-based diet for personal health reasons. There is absolutely nothing anyone can do or say that would be antagonistic or misunderstanding about your situation. You're being honest, and then he or she can be prepared.

On the Fly

If you must grab-and-go, there are definitely better options out there than deep-fried onion rings. Most fast-food restaurants have salads, and some have veggie chili and soups. A better option would be to run into a grocery store and grab an avocado roll or some fresh fruit. In *The Kind Diet*, Alicia Silverstone discusses these choices. She writes that she just simply tries to make good decisions when confronted with a situation such as eating on the go. She gives the example that even if she's stuck going to a 7-Eleven for grub, she can always walk out with raw sunflower seeds and an apple juice, which would be a whole lot better than most of the alternatives offered there.[247]

Be a Girl Scout! (Be Prepared)

The following foods are ones that should be removed from the diet of anyone who wants or needs to recalibrate their bodies from the inside out, especially for the first few weeks of detoxification:

Meat, dairy, processed sugar, processed foods, anything genetically modified, caffeine and alcohol all should go in order to achieve the best results in the shortest amount of time. These foods harm; you need to begin consuming foods that heal. The exception to sugar is fruit. If you can't live without red wine (I totally get you), reintroduce it after this initial period. If you can, purchase an organic label.

When you do this, the first week or so will be tense. You might experience headaches, constipation, diarrhea, and irritableness. These are symptoms of detoxification, which you will definitely be going through. Sugar (in particular) is a drug, and your body will be initially resistant to its disappearance. To aid in your successful accomplishment of the task of truly removing these disease-provoking foods from your diet, simply take anything that falls into the "nix" category, box it up, and give it away. This is to prevent temporary relapses when the going gets tough. Open your refrigerator, and take a good look at what's in there. Imagine me standing behind you. What would I be suggesting that you chuck? If you live with others who plan on still consuming these foods, then try and create a separate area of the pantry for yourself. You can stock this area with good foods that you will shop for shortly. Use the Pantry Prerequisites (page 184) and

Meal Ideas (Page 190) sections in this book to get an idea of foods you can consume. Prepare a grocery list, and shop for items listed there.

With regards to giving up meat and animal products: there are tons of substitutes out there (you can swap your mayonnaise for Vegannaise, and your butter for Earth's Balance Buttery Spread), and there is no reason to keep these in your diet, nutritionally speaking. They will only do you harm, and your body needs a break. Also, there are a great many people out there who are lactose intolerant. By not consuming dairy products for at least a month, you will notice if they bother you afterwards. You might be so used to feeling stomach pain that you can't decipher where it originated from. Dairy's a tricky little bugger!

It's also very important to begin consuming at least eight glasses of purified water and/or peppermint, ginger, fennel, or chamomile herbal teas every day. Nothing else will hydrate you better. Maybe experiment with some pure coconut water. (Read the ingredients and make certain that it's only coconut water; no added sugar.) Again, try and refrain from caffeine and alcohol, because this will inevitably aggravate your digestive system, and slow down the healing process. If you are super brave, start juicing in the morning. This is a fabulous way to kick-start this plan, and fresh, raw juices on an empty stomach will help the detoxification process. Just a word of caution: if you aren't used to consuming a lot of raw vegetables and fruits, then don't start with the green juice. Slowly work up to that one by juicing the other recipes for a couple of weeks first, and then try adding the green juice to your menu. It's the best for you, but it can cause alot of excitability in your digestive parts.

Add some whole grains and beans into the mix. Whole grains, beans, fruits, veggies, water, herbal tea, and juices are what you should be consuming a good 80% of the time. You will see a huge change within two weeks if you do this, and not only digestively speaking. Kelly, who told her colitis story earlier in this book, lost thirteen pounds in her first three weeks on this plan! Ideally, you should be consuming five small meals daily, and they need to be equally spaced apart. You need to give yourself enough time to sit down, chew well, and be relaxed while you eat. Do not drink any liquids while eating; it will only interfere with proper digestion. Wait for about half an hour after a meal to drink anything.

Begin your new venture by writing up a weekly meal plan for yourself. If you are in the middle of a flare-up, then foods should be relatively bland in the first two weeks, and in theory, easy to digest. You should also be taking probiotics upon waking up. This will help reintroduce good bacteria to your gut, and improve intestinal flora. Remember that organics are better for you. You will want to rid your body of the chemicals and genetically modified ingredients that are probably running around, partying hard in your colon. Include tons of whole, sprouted grains, fresh vegetables (including sprouts), and beans. Fruits and nuts are great too. Also, if you are truly planning on taking the full-on vegan route, I recommend taking a B12 supplement at least two or three times a week.

There are several ways in which you can make this food transition easier for yourself. Instead of thinking that you must give up all of your favorite foods, just make small changes to them in order to make them meat-free, and more whole. For example, if you like hotdogs and fries, try a veggie dog on a whole wheat bun, and side it with roasted yams. Super yummy! Or, instead of beef tacos, substitute the beef for black beans. Just tweaking your favorite foods can help you accomplish this dietary change. Try the meat substitutes, and then transition to making your own at home. (Homemade veggie burgers are the best!) Try buying sprouts from the grocery store first, then go ahead and sprout your own when you feel comfortable. Baby steps, right?

Keep an open mind. This might seem restrictive, but it's really what you make it out to be. Restriction is what is going on with your situation now; this plan is all about freedom. Many people know that they should be eating this way, but they don't really give it proper consideration because they assume it will be really difficult. It's not! It's fun, and it forces you to try new foods and become more creative with your cooking. Also, remember why you are doing this. This plan is for better quality of life. It will eliminate many if not all of your digestive disorder's symptoms, and treat the root of the digestive problem itself. This is for long-term wellness. There is no way for this diet to be bad for you—its good, clean, whole food. This is for you, because you deserve to live without chronic pain. I know what this lifestyle change is about, and I am confident that it can vastly improve your entire life. It's been three years for me, and I'm still learning new things every day. It takes time, but it's worth it. I'm pain free, and so is everyone who shared their story in this book. We all treated ourselves without drugs or surgeries. We simply healed ourselves with food.

Hopefully by now, you're revved and inspired, and ready to go. The information in the last chapter is a general outline to provide you with an idea of how to begin this lifestyle game-changer. This plan is tailored to take into account all of the goings-on of a toxic, stressed, run-down digestive system. By removing such clutter as bad food, chemicals, non-nutritive drinks, stress, insomnia, and as a by-product, excess fat from your life, you will be a new, very happy person. I cannot emphasize enough that if you follow this plan, you will absolutely attain freedom from that which has been holding you down. You will only feel better, and it will happen very quickly. Hooray!

Question: Which foods are you most interested in trying? Do you eat any of these foods already? Highlight what you need to remember, and look forward to implementing these ideas as a way to build the new you! Tear down your current pantry, then make a new food list to build it back up with the building blocks to digestive success. Write down as many yummy-sounding ingredients down as you can, and go rock the grocery store. It's a liberating feeling to be able to leave your old foods on the curb, and fill your pantry with new and interesting substitutes. Shopping with your eyes open is an activity too few of us participate in.

Chapter 12

Get Healthy, Feel Beautiful

"Love the life you live. Live the life you love."[248]

—Bob Marley

Everyone is responsible for making their own decisions regarding how to live their lives, and food is at the forefront of living. It is a very personal subject, because it literally makes us who we are. Food directly contributes to how we feel, what we look like, how much energy we have, how well we sleep, our power to fight off infection and disease, our longevity, and more.

My personal stance on the issue of "to be" or "not to be" vegetarian was originally one of mixed feelings, and I think that was because I didn't like the label. This is how I came to the conclusion that I wanted to be a "plant-based" eater or a "plant-strong eater." eater. Not "vegetarian" or "vegan." My diet is made up of mostly plant-based foods (I would say about 95%), but I also eat a little bit of wild, fresh fish every now and then, and maybe a little goat cheese on my salad when I feel that I need to indulge. The difference between eating these items for me, and eating a piece of steak, is that I now understand what my body can handle and what it can't, in terms of digesting the food I supply it with. I can handle a bit of salmon and goat cheese, but my stomach would divorce me (that's literally what it feels like it's trying to do) if I got anywhere near a hamburger. After many years and far too much gut ache, I finally know my limits. The goal for you is to figure out the same, and if you begin by ridding yourself of all foods that could possibly cause concern and/or inflammation, and just eat simply and mindfully, you will get to know your body. You don't have to live by a label that defines who you are, or what you eat. Just be you, only better. Be the *best* version of yourself. Eat what makes you feel amazing, what makes your soul sing, and what makes your gut sigh with relief over the cessation of chronic pain.

"The only person who likes change is a newborn, and it's natural, it's human nature. Anywhere you go, 99% of the people are eating incorrectly. The numbers are against you, and it's very hard for those 99% to look at you in the 1% and say, 'Yes, he's right, we are all wrong'."[249]
—Dr. Caldwell Esselstyn, JR, MD, *The China Study*

It's sometimes very confusing that there can be such a general lack of enthusiasm for something that obviously results in better health for everyone, regardless of age, gender, and previous medical history.

Let's use an analogy. Say you are a realtor, who has recently stumbled upon a remarkable, yet fairly obvious and simple way of selling homes more efficiently and effectively. When you use your new selling method, your sales triple. Now, say you share this information with your sales team, because you want them to thrive too. Everyone wants to make more money, right? Imagine getting uncomfortable feedback from your team right away; they don't even want to try it, despite your assurance of better sales. That would be really bewildering. They have nothing to lose and everything to gain, but they still want to stick to their same old sales method, which only makes them a fraction of what they could make if they ventured out and tried something proven to increase their income.

Do you choose familiarity and mediocrity, or do you trust in others' experience, and reap the rewards? Do you decide to make considerably less than what you could, or double your income? Would you rather be half sick, or genuinely and undeniably healthy?

The day after I decided to adopt this lifestyle change, somebody close to me that I was conversing with about my new dietary venture said, "Just don't feed your kids that crap." I was pretty shocked, and a little hurt. I felt as though I had just made the best lifestyle choice of my twenty-nine years, and was already getting grief for it. This was to be the first situation of many in which my defenses were raised and my decision reinforced. I'm sort of contrary like that. If you get similar reactions from people who are close to you, please do not become discouraged. Take it as a challenge.

By showing a good example when it comes to eating healthy food, educating yourself about the food industry as we *don't* know it, and exemplifying how conscious eating can eradicate the most common digestive disorders, hopefully your friends and family will understand why you gave up or altered some of your favorite foods, and what it has meant for your health and quality of life. Perhaps they might eventually consider adopting a plant-based diet themselves! It's about opening each other's eyes about what the food we choose to eat means to our health, the welfare of our fellow sentient beings, and the effects it has on our environment and planet. I think these are important considerations to pass on to each other, and to our future generations.

In early 2012, the University of California went public with a study that they feel warrants the taxation of sugar.[250] My husband

and I watched this story unfold on the news together, and he thought that the notion was ridiculous, because people are intelligent, and should be able to make up their own minds and know when enough sugar is enough, without another intrusive, government tax.

While I do agree with my husband's opinion, I also forecast that we are going to see alot more of these broad accusations and conclusions on single nutrients aimed towards developing better nutrition for the general population in the next decade or so. When governments accepted that tobacco smoke was indeed deadly, they taxed tobacco to over double the former price per pack in order to deter people from buying and smoking cigarettes. When studies began bubbling to the surface about the harmful effects of food being stored in plastic containers, and the use of the chemical BPA, we ditched them for old-school glass ones. Now that organic food is becoming more available and mainstream, and more information is being provided about it, we have slowly come to accept that the alternative to eating organic is buy food that has been genetically modified and grown using harmful chemicals.

That's a gut-wrenching alternative!

I believe, without a single doubt, that eventually we will all have to admit that sugar is terrible for us, and we will have to pay a higher price to consume it, but it is my most sincere hope that in the very near future, we will collectively begin to understand that mainstream, factory-farmed animal products, genetically modified foods, and foods that are riddled with chemical additives are not helping us in any way, either. I am very optimistic that when enough noise is created about the disease-provoking effects that these foods have on our bodies, the devastating results that factory farming has on the environment, and the undeniably frustrating outcome of grain being diverted to livestock instead of being shared with fellow human beings, that we can all finally admit that a plant-based diet is the only viable and sustainable solution to these substantial and growing problems.

Our western diet is awful, and it's the largest contributor to our digestion being awful, too. It contains far too much animal meat, dairy, processed food, and chemical additives, while encouraging the consumption of far too few whole grains, raw vegetables, and just plain nourishment. We also rely too heavily on medications and surgeries to repair our ailments, instead of looking to what we literally need in order to live and prosper, which is simply good, fresh, whole, and healing food.

We really are what we eat. If we consume fresh produce and whole grains, we will feel young, vibrant and be whole. If we fill our bodies with chemicals, animal proteins, and fast food, we will become toxic, overweight, and proceed to get sick at an alarming rate.

"Food shouldn't need to be irradiated to be safe. Animals shouldn't need to be pumped full of antibiotics. We shouldn't be ingesting food that is making us sick and depressed. We shouldn't be living on cocktails of drugs or weight-loss pills. Animals shouldn't be bred to grow so big so fast that their joints can't support their weight. And we shouldn't have people suffering from malnutrition in this land of plenty."[251]

—Gene Baur, *Farm Sanctuary*

We know change is forthcoming because of the growing demand for organic food and naturally-raised animals, and people all over are beginning to pay attention to these more readily available products, and learning about the health benefits that they offer. It's a giant learning curve, but we are all going to get there. Why not give yourself a more substantial chance at success on the digestive front, and start now? You don't have to be in pain anymore—don't accept a mediocre life. You deserve better, so start treating yourself as if you do. Start thinking food-forward! Will that lunch you ordered help or hinder your body? How will eating it make you feel after? These questions matter, because your happiness matters. Your life matters. Don't waste time feeling sub-par!

We have to open our eyes and ears and be morally at peace with the decisions that we make in regards to an issue we face several times every day: what to eat. You are your own best advocate for change, and you deserve to experience wellness that you may have long ago given up on. There are so many reasons to adopt a whole food, plant-based diet. Pick one, or three, or all, and go for it! Borrowing John Robbins' words of wisdom:

"If you eat consciously, exercise regularly, and seek to enjoy every precious moment of your life, you won't be another one of the people who end up lamenting, 'If I had known I was going to live this long, I would have taken better care of myself'."[252]

Here's the bottom line: there are millions of people out there living every single day in digestive unease. For some, it's completely debilitating and for others it's merely annoying. No matter where you lie in regards to this spectrum, it's treatable, and treatable by *you*. We rely too heavily on medical doctors who are not adequately trained on nutrition to give us advice that is largely trial and error, and little of it addresses the root of the problem: food. We need to quit masking our symptoms and start treating the actual issue. By empowering ourselves to holistically and simply repair our digestive dysfunction from the inside out (ironically by altering that from which the outside gets in), we can take back control of our lives in a way that leaves no room for side-effects, expensive treatments, surgeries, consultations, or wasted time or money in any fashion.

You picked up this book for a reason. You are either thinking of making a major dietary change, or you already have and you need some further encouragement. Although digestive disease runs in my family, I don't feel that anyone has to play the genetic lottery. Genetics only account for a very small percentage of your risk of these diseases, which means you can overcome the odds through lifestyle; mainly diet. Whatever your reason for investigating a plant-based diet, I can assure you that eating plants and forgoing meat will help you feel light, lose weight, clear your skin, ease your pains, help the planet, feed the hungry, and save some animals. What you're about to embark upon will make you happy, from the inside, out. Own it. Love it. This is the start of an even more amazing you, and a healthier, longer life for everyone who decides that a whole food, plant-based diet just makes the most sense.

Cheers to fabulous health!

Question: Are you ready for a happy, healthy gut?

Chapter 13

The Recalibration Plan and Kick-Ass Recipes

Adopting a new way to prepare and think about food is going to be fabulous, and you're going to be amazed. Experiment with cooking something new, and definitely invest in a few fabulous vegetarian or vegan recipe books. They can be awesome and inspiring and very helpful in the task of breathing new life into your old food habits. I provide the names of my favorite recipe books in the References section at the end of this book.

This is a lifestyle make-over, and that includes improving your whole mind, body, and soul. Attend a yoga class. Go get some organic aromatherapy oil, or lavender scented soy candles. Breathe them in! You're going to love being free of stomach pain. You will naturally rehydrate, lose weight, and clear up your skin. People will notice and ask you for your secret. Share it! We need to pass on this message of encouragement to one another. Digestive problems are terrible to live with—I know you know. Adopting this type of plan also means ridding yourself of the common "western diet," which in turn means that you are going to lower your risk of developing any of the chronic diseases in that category, including diabetes, coronary heart disease, hypertension, certain cancers (colon cancer, certainly), obesity and more. I'm so excited for you!

The Recalibration Plan Made Simple

You've made it to this point! Now it will get easier. This is a comprehensive review of what you need to do to begin your days in Digestive Bliss Town:

- Decide that you want to feel awesome. (Page 137)
- Clean out your pantry. (Page 204)
- Make a meal plan for the week, every week. Follow it. (Page 190)
- Shop for foods that will help you stick to your meal plan. Use the list of foods in the "pantry prerequisite" section. (Page 184)
- Make sure you read the ingredients on what you buy. Try and purchase foods that possess only a few ingredients. (Page 134)
- Remember to stick to the perimeter of the store, for the most part. (Page 135)
- Drink more water, and make sure it's filtered. (Page 127)
- Buy organic food as much as possible. (Page 135)
- Know your superfoods. (Page 141)
- Eat the rainbow. (Page 143)
- Discover if food combining works for you. (Page 148)
- Buy foods that are locally grown. (Page 151)
- Ferment, sprout, and juice. (Pages 151-157)
- Invest in some new kitchenware to help motivate you to start cooking. (Page 157)

- Reduce stress. (Page 162)
- Know how to react to a flare-up. (Page 163)
- Consider taking natural supplements. (Page 164)
- Make sure you are moving your bowels. (Page 170)
- Slow down and relax. (Page 162)
- Try Yoga. (Page 166)
- Begin taking Vitamin B12 if you plan on going completely vegan. (Page 181)
- Invest in some new, inspiring recipe books. (Page 239)

Try and Avoid:

- Animal products. (A common running theme–no page number necessary!)
- Irradiated food. (Page 92)
- GMOs. (Page 94)
- Chemicals. (Page 111)
- Processed food. (Page 105)
- Sugar. (Page 120)
- Caffeine and alcohol. (Page 175)

Use the meal plan on the following page to provide yourself with an example on how to structure your new eating schedule. Feel free to change it completely, or follow it exactly. It's your choice; the guide is just an easy reference to get you started. It's also been created in such a way as to make it easy to follow, even if you are working a nine-to-five kind of stint. Everything from Monday to Friday can easily be prepared ahead of time and brought to work, while the weekend meals are a little more creative and better suited for having access to your own kitchen. Remember that aside from the meals listed on the next few pages, you need to make sure that you are drinking lots of filtered water throughout the day. Include two or three cups of herbal tea, and try and aim for a total of sixty- four ounces of clear fluids a day.

One-Week Recalibration Meal Plan

Monday

7am: Stretch, probiotics, Beginner Juice. (See recipe on page 156)

8am: 1 cup "Om" Oatmeal. (See recipe on page 216)

10am: Apple with 1 tbsp. almond butter, herbal tea.

12pm: Whole wheat wrap with raw veggies and hummus, (see recipe on page 224) carrot sticks. Add fermented veggies to the wrap if you feel brave.

3pm: 6 green olives, herbal tea.

6pm: Superfood Salad. (See recipe on page 217)

8pm: Herbal tea, 10 minutes of stretching and quiet, conscious breathing.

Tuesday

7am: Stretch, probiotics, anti-inflammatory juice. (See recipe on page 156)

8am: Superfood Smoothie. (See recipe on page 213)

10am: ½ cup soy yogurt, 4 strawberries, herbal tea, vitamin B12 capsule.

12pm: Garden salad, ¼ cup mixed and raw sunflower and pumpkin seeds, dressing of choice.

3pm: Apple, herbal tea.

6pm: Love Soup. (See recipe on page 218)

8pm: Herbal tea, 10 minutes of stretching and quiet, conscious breathing.

Wednesday

7am: Stretch, probiotics, Breakfast Juice. (See recipe on page 156)

8am: 1 slice sprouted grain bread, 1 tbsp. almond butter, 1 pear.

10am: 2 celery stalks, 1 tbsp. tahini, herbal tea.

12pm: Leftover soup.

3pm: 10 raw almonds, herbal tea.

6pm: Quinoa Salad. (See recipe on page 217)

8pm: Herbal tea, 10 minutes of stretching and quiet, conscious breathing.

Thursday

7am: Stretch, probiotics, Green Juice. (See recipe on page 156)

8am: Blonde Muesli. (See recipe on page 216)

10am: ½ cup soy yogurt, ½ cup blueberries, herbal tea, vitamin B12 capsule.

12pm: Greek Pita. (See recipe on page 216)

3pm: Raw carrot sticks, 1 tbsp. tahini, herbal tea.

6pm: Vegalicious Chili. (See recipe on page 219)

8pm: Herbal tea, 10 minutes of stretching and quiet, conscious breathing.

Friday

7am: Stretch, probiotics, Intermediate Juice. (See recipe on page 156)

8am: Strawberry-Banana Smoothie, ¼ cup raw almonds. (See recipe on page 212)

10am: Pear, 1 tbsp. almond butter, herbal tea.

12pm: Leftover chili.

3pm: ½ avocado topped with Fresh Salsa, herbal tea. (See recipe on page 214)

6pm: ½ cup brown rice, 1 cup steamed veggies, 2 ounces tofu (organic and firm), 1 tbsp. tamari.

8pm: Herbal tea, 10 minutes of stretching and quiet, conscious breathing.

Saturday

7am: Stretch, probiotics, Beginner Juice. (See recipe on page 156)

8am: ½ cup cooked quinoa, 1 banana sliced on top, splash of unsweetened almond milk.

10am: Small bowl of fruit salad, 6-8 pecans, herbal tea, vitamin B12 capsule.

12pm: Rainbow Chard and Beet Salad. (See recipe on page 217)

3pm: Kale chips (full bunch), herbal tea. (See recipe on page 217)

6pm: Super Easy Vegan Tacos. (See recipe on page 220)

8pm: Herbal tea, 10 minutes of stretching and quiet, conscious breathing.

Sunday

7am: Stretch, probiotics, Anti-Inflammatory Juice. (See recipe on page 156)

8am: Leftover fruit salad, 10 raw walnuts, dollop of soy yogurt, 1 tbsp. chia seeds.

10am: 1 slice sprouted grain bread, 1 tbsp. hummus, handful of assorted sprouts, herbal tea.

12pm: Amy's Organic Lentil Soup (whole can).

3pm: Pear, herbal tea.

6pm: 2 Stuffed Portabella Mushroomss. (See recipe on page 218)

8pm: Herbal tea, 10 minutes of stretching and quiet, conscious breathing.

Restorative Recipes

The following recipes include those for the One-Week Recalibration Meal Plan, and more. Feel free to make them to your heart's content!

Liquids

Strawberry-Banana Smoothie-serves two

My family's favorite. Who can improve on strawberries and bananas?

1½ cups of water   12 frozen strawberries

2 bananas   20 raw walnuts

Combine all ingredients except walnuts in blender. Blend for one minute. Pour into two tall glasses, and top with walnuts. Substitute the water for unsweetened soy milk if you would like a more calorie-dense smoothie. (Meal replacement)

Superfood Smoothie-serves one

This smoothie is absolutely teeming with vitamins. It makes a fab lunch replacement!

1 cup of filtered water	1 tbsp. chia seeds
2 cups fresh spinach	Agave syrup to taste
¾ cup frozen blueberries	

Combine all ingredients into blender in this order listed above. Blend for 1 minute. Drink up!

Green Smoothie-serves one

½ honeydew melon	1 cucumber
1 chunk ginger	1 cup of ice
1 pear	

Juice the ginger, pear, and cucumber. Pour into blender, and add melon. Blend until smooth. Place ice into a tall glass, then add smoothie. Drink ice cold.

Strawberry-Mint Summer Cocktail-serves two

This pretty drink is crazy refreshing.

1 can club soda	10 fresh mint leaves
Filtered water	1 lime
6 sliced organic strawberries	Agave syrup to taste

Using 2 tall glasses, fill half way with ice. Pour half a can of club soda into each. Divide strawberries and mint leaves, and place half in each glass. Fill to 1 inch from top with filtered water. Add 1 tbsp. agave syrup to each glass. Mix well. Squeeze fresh lime juice on top of each drink. Enjoy!

Note: Rub mint leaves between your fingers before placing in glasses. This will help release the flavor.

Nibbles
Kale Chips-serves two

My absolute favorite way to eat kale. I even have my neighbors hooked!

1 bunch fresh kale	Sea salt to taste
Pinch of nutritional yeast	

Set oven to 350 degrees Fahrenheit. Wash and dry kale; rip into pieces. Spread the kale out on a cookie sheet in a single layer. Grind sea salt lightly over top. Bake for approximately 8 minutes, until edges of kale are crisp-looking. Remove from heat and place on cooling rack. Evenly sprinkle nutritional yeast over the kale. Eat within a couple of hours.

Fresh Salsa-makes two cups

12 grape tomatoes	Small bunch of cilantro
1 yellow bell pepper	1 lime
1 small jalapeño pepper	1 cup black beans
1 small red onion	

Combine peppers and onion into food processor. Pulse until roughly chopped. Add tomatoes and cilantro. Pulse until tomatoes are diced to your size preference. Add juice from lime and black beans. Stir by hand. Serve with organic tortilla chips, or as a topper for half an avocado.

Chocolate Chia Pudding-serves one

A great friend of mine got me hooked on this one. It makes a yummy snack, and even the kids like it.

1 cup chocolate almond milk	3 tbsp. chia seeds
	3 tbsp. raw coconut

Stir chia seeds into milk, on and off, for about five minutes. Seeds need to be evenly distributed in the milk. Cover and refrigerate overnight. In morning, sprinkle coconut on top and eat. High-fiber pudding for breakfast!

Apple Snack-serves one

This snack is super easy and fast to make, and it is high in energy and raw goodness.

1 apple
1 tbsp. almond or peanut
    butter
2 tbsp. rolled oats

Core apple, and cut in half. Fill each half with ½ tbsp. of nut butter. Sprinkle oats on top. Easy snack!

Holy Guacamole-makes one cup

2 avocados
1 roma tomato
1 garlic clove
1 cup cilantro
1 lime
Pinch of sea salt

Combine all ingredients in food processor or blender. Blend until slightly chunky. Serve with organic tortilla chips, or as a dip for fresh veggies.

Nori Roll-serves one

Why go for Japanese, when you can make your own? The flavors in this light lunch are delicious!

1 sheet nori
¼ cup julienned carrots and
    cucumber
½ avocado sliced vertically
¼ cup cooked brown rice
¼ cup tamari for dipping

Wet nori, and place on smooth surface. Place brown rice on top, then veggies. Carefully roll into a roll, wrap-style. Dip in tamari for each bite.

Meals

"Om" Oatmeal-serves two

This breakfast will keep your tummy full for hours, and is high in protein and yumminess.

1 cup rolled oats	Filtered water
2 tbsp. hemp hearts	Pumpkin and sunflower
¼ cup dried dates	seeds to garnish
1 tbsp. ground flaxseed	

Combine the first four ingredients into a stainless steel pot. Fill with filtered water to just cover oat mixture. Cook on low-medium heat until water is absorbed; about 5 minutes. Stir a few times throughout. Remove from stove and scoop into two bowls. Top with pumpkin and sunflower seeds.

Blonde Muesli-serves one

This pretty breakfast is magic for your taste buds. It's easy to make, and super nutritious.

½ pear sliced thinly	1 tbsp. white chia seeds
2 tbsp. wheat germ	½ cup unsweetened almond
¼ cup shredded coconut	milk
½ cup rolled oats	Cinnamon to taste

Layer ingredients in the above order in a bowl. Eat immediately!

Greek Pita-serves two

A very filling lunch! Everybody loves a make-your-own kinda dish, and this meal does not disappoint.

1 whole wheat pita	¼ diced red onion
½ cup cooked brown rice	¼ diced cucumber
½ cup chickpeas	4 tbsp hummus (recipe on
1 diced roma tomato	page 224)

Cut pita in half; gently open both halves without tearing bottoms. Layer remaining ingredients in pita in the order they are listed. So yummy!

Rainbow Chard-Beet Salad-serves two

This is a pretty and perfect salad for a fall or winter meal. The warmth of the rice and roasted beet create cozy flavors and textures that make you feel snuggly.

4 rainbow chard leaves	½ cup raw walnuts
2 medium-sized beets	¼ cup raw sunflower seeds
½ cup cooked brown rice	Dressing of your choice
1 cup chickpeas or lentils	

Set oven at 325 degrees Fahrenheit. Clean beets and wrap individually with foil. Place in oven-safe dish, and roast for 30-40 minutes until they are easily diced. Set aside to cool until just warm. Cook rice. Set aside to cool until just warm. Wash and dry chard, remove rib, rip into pieces, and divide onto two plates. Dice beets, and divide beets, rice, and beans, and place on top of chard. Add walnuts and seeds, then drizzle dressing on top. Serve immediately while still warm.

Superfood Salad-serves two

This light, summery salad is a sister to the smoothie version.

1 bunch spinach	¼ cup pumpkin seeds
1 avocado	¼ cup walnuts
½ cup blueberries	Dressing of your choice

Wash and dry spinach, rip into pieces and plate. Add diced avocado, blueberries, seeds, and nuts. Drizzle White Dressing to taste.

Quinoa Salad-serves six

This salad is perfect to make for dinner, and then bring to work for lunch the next day. Super high in protein *and* deliciousness.

1 cup quinoa

2 cups vegetable stock

½ cucumber

12 grape tomatoes

6 basil leaves

1 can drained and rinsed
  chickpeas

1 tbsp. fresh pressed garlic

Combine quinoa and stock and bring to a boil. Turn heat down to low, and simmer for about 15 minutes. Remove from burner and place lid on top, letting it sit for another 5 minutes. Remove lid and cool. Once quinoa reaches room temperature, dice cucumber, and cut grape tomatoes in half. Cut basil leaves into thin strips. Combine all ingredients into large bowl and mix well. Keeps for a couple of days in the fridge.

Stuffed Portabella Mushrooms-serves two

This is a great dinner meal for its presentation qualities alone! Filling and robust, this is one vegan entree that your omnivorous friends will want to make themselves.

4 portabella mushrooms

1 small fennel bulb

2 tbsp. sundried tomatoes

2 garlic cloves

½ yellow onion

2 celery stalks

¼ cup Daiya

Set oven at 350 degrees Fahrenheit. Wash mushrooms, and pull off stems. Dice fennel, onion, celery, and mushroom stems. Heat frying pan, and add garlic, diced fennel, onion, and celery. Cook until they are just softened. Remove from heat, and add sundried tomatoes, diced mushroom stems, and Daiya. Mix well. Scoop ¼ of mixture into cavity of each mushroom. Bake for 20 minutes, or until heated through. Serve two stuffed mushrooms per person.

Love Soup-serves six

This soup is so nutritious, you can feel the love slip right down into your belly! Great for cooler nights.

½ cup dried lentils

6-8 roma tomatoes

1 tetra pack of organic
vegetable broth

2 celery stalks

1 white onion

1 fennel bulb

3 carrots

1 leek

½ cup brown, sprouted rice

1 tbsp. onion powder

1 tsp. garlic salt

1 tbsp. dried basil

1 tbsp. dried parsley

1 tbsp. dried oregano

Salt and pepper to taste

Soak lentils overnight, then rinse, drain, and set aside. Blend tomatoes in foods processor until liquidly. Pour liquid into a standard-sized crock pot. Add vegetable broth. Throw celery, onion, fennel, and carrots in food processor. Blend until desired size. Add to crock pot. Chop leek, then add it and the dry rice to crock pot mixture. Add all herbs, and mix well. Cover and let cook on low for about six hours. Before serving, add lentils and mix well. Serve hot, with a warmed, sprouted grain bun.

Vegalicious Chili-serves six

My husband prefers this dish without the vegan ground round, but I prefer it with. Your choice!

1 large can diced tomatoes

1 can red kidney beans

1 cup filtered water

1 package of vegan ground
round (optional)

2 carrots

1 green pepper

1 onion

2 cloves garlic

1 tbsp. chili powder

1 tbsp. red pepper chili
flakes

1 tbsp. onion powder

1 tsp. garlic salt

2 bay leaves

½ cup Daiya

Drain and rinse beans well. Combine onion, green pepper, carrots, and garlic in food processor. Process for about 7-8 seconds on high. Combine mixture with beans, tomatoes, water, spices, and bay leaves in crock pot. Cook on high for two hours, or low for 6 hours. Stir occasionally. Just before serving, break up ground round and mix into crock pot well. Remove bay leaves, and serve hot. Top with Daiya.

Super Easy Vegan Tacos-serves three

This is one of my fave meals. I love messy eats, and this one is up there with the best of them.

6 hard taco shells

1 cup black beans

½ small head of chopped raw cabbage

1 cup Fresh Salsa (recipe on page 214)

2 tbsp. chili powder

1 avocado, diced

1 lime

¼ cup raw sunflower seeds

Combine black beans, salsa, and chili powder in one bowl. Combine cabbage, lime juice, sunflower seeds, and avocado in another bowl. Fill your shell half way with bean mixture, and the rest of the way with cabbage mixture. Bon Appetite!

Note: Fresh Salsa already contains black beans, but for this dish you will want to add extra. Hence the additional cup of beans . . .

Marie's Vegan Thai Red Curry-serves four

This Thai dish is to die for. It's completely vegan, and totally amazing.

2 cans unsweetened coconut milk

2 tbsp. curry paste

1 yellow onion

3 garlic cloves

3 yellow potatoes

1 bunch cauliflower florets

1 can bamboo shoots

1 to 2 red bell peppers

1 package firm tofu, cut into ½-inch cubes

Dice onion and potatoes, mince garlic, cut peppers into long, thin strips, break apart cauliflower into pieces, and cut tofu into one-inch cubes. Set aside. Spoon out half of one of the cans of coconut

milk, incorporating any thicker part and bring to a gentle boil over medium heat. Cook stirring occasionally, until milk releases its sweet fragrance, about three minutes. Add curry paste and cook for three minutes more, mashing, scraping and stirring often to soften the paste and combine it with the coconut milk. Add onion and garlic, stirring gently to coat with curry paste. Sauté for 5 minutes. Add remaining 1½ cans coconut milk, tofu, potatoes, cauliflower and bamboo shoots. Combine well, and bring to an active boil. Reduce heat to maintain a gentle boil and simmer for 15 minutes, stirring occasionally. Add red peppers and stir gently. Cook for 5 more minutes, until peppers are cooked but not too soft. Serve over rice.
*Thanks to Marie Arnold for this contribution

Eggplant Lasagne-serves six

This hearty lasagne is major comfort food, and super flavorful. The chia seeds act as a binding agent in place of egg.

1 package whole wheat lasagne noodles	1 bunch spinach
4 cups diced tomatoes	¼ cup chia seeds
1 eggplant	¼ cup ground flaxseed
1 onion	4 garlic cloves
2 carrots	1 tbsp. oregano
4 celery stalks	1 tbsp. red chili pepper flakes
1 cup mushrooms	1 tbsp. onion powder
1 cup Daiya	

Set oven at 350 degrees Fahrenheit, and wash all produce. Combine onion, carrots, celery, and mushrooms in your food processor. Process on high for about 5 seconds. Combine mixture with diced tomatoes, flaxseed, and all spices in stainless steel pot. Simmer, covered, for 30 minutes. Meanwhile, cook noodles until half done. (Still firm) Thinly slice eggplant length-wise about 8 times. Sparingly coat baking dish with avocado oil. Beginning with the noodles, cover the bottom in a single layer. Then, stir chia seeds into sauce, and spoon half the sauce over the noodles. Lay eggplant in single layer over top, and then cover generously with spinach. Repeat with noodles, sauce, eggplant, spinach, noodles, and then end with sauce. Sprinkle with Daiya, and bake for 45 minutes to an hour. Let cool for 10 minutes before serving.

Sweets

Cocoa Energy Bars-makes approximately fifteen bars

1 cup rolled oats	¼ cup raw cocoa powder
½ cup pumpkin seeds	2 tbsp. chia seeds
½ cup dried cranberries	2 tbsp. flax seeds
¼ cup sunflower seeds	1 cup brown rice syrup
¼ cup walnut pieces	¼ cup maple syrup

Combine all ingredients in bowl and mix well, until sticky and evenly coated. Line 9x13 baking pan with parchment paper. Pour mixture into pan, and pat down firmly. Cover with foil, and refrigerate overnight. Cut into bars.

Summer Crumble-serves six

4 cups of assorted frozen or fresh fruit	½ cup brown sugar
	½ cup Earth's Balance
1 cup rolled oats	Buttery Spread
½ cup whole wheat flour	1 tbsp. cinnamon

Preheat oven to 350 degrees Fahrenheit. Toss fruit with cinnamon and pour into non-stick 8x8 baking pan. Combine oats, flour, sugar, and butter substitute. Pour over fruit, and pat down gently to form crust. Bake for 45 minutes. Let cool for 10 minutes, then serve hot.

Poached Pears-serves six

6 organic pears (not overly ripe)	2 tbsp. raw cane sugar
	2 tbsp. cinnamon

1 tsp. cloves   Organic plain soy yogurt

Preheat oven to 350 degrees Fahrenheit. Core pears and cut in half. Place a small amount of water into a baking pan, so that it is about ½ deep. Place pears in baking pan, meat-side up (skin-side down). Combine sugar, cinnamon, and cloves. Divide evenly, and sprinkle mixture over each pear. Bake for 30 minutes. Turn oven to broil, and cook pears for another 5 minutes, or until tops begin to brown. (Keep an eye! The sugar burns fast.) Remove from oven, and let cool slightly. Fill cavity with a dollop of soy yogurt and serve immediately, 2 halves each.

Dark Chocolate Fruit Kabobs-serves four

½ cantaloupe, cut into chunks

16 strawberries, halved

2 bananas, cut into small chunks

16 seedless grapes, whole

1 bar of organic, dark chocolate

8 bamboo skewers

Slide fruit evenly onto skewers, about 8 pieces per skewer. Melt dark chocolate using a double broiler on the stove. Arrange kabobs on plate, then using a small metal spoon, drizzle melted chocolate over kabobs evenly. Serve immediately.

Extras

Tahini Dipping Sauce-serves four

2 garlic cloves
½ cup basil or cilantro
½ tsp. sea salt
2 tbsp. lemon juice
½ cup water
½ cup tahini paste

Blend garlic, herbs, salt, and lemon juice in food processor. Add water and tahini, and process until smooth. Use for a spread in sandwiches, burgers, and wraps.

Hummus-makes one and a half cups

Great for a sandwich spread, veggie dip, and more.

1 can rinsed and drained
   chickpeas
2 cloves garlic
½ cup water

2 tbsp. tahini
2 tbsp. lemon juice
½ tsp. cumin

Blend all ingredients in food processor. Enjoy!

White Poppy Dressing-makes approximately 1 cup

½ cup unsweetened almond
   milk
½ tbsp. poppy seeds
¼ cup minced shallots
¼ cup green onion

2 cloves garlic
⅛ cup white wine vinegar
Pinch of black pepper
Pinch of sea salt

Combine all ingredients in food processor and blend well. Keeps in refrigerator for about a week. Shake well before each use.

Miso Dressing-makes half a cup

¼ cup miso
2 tbsp. rice vinegar
2 tbsp. tamari

2 tbsp. water
1 tsp. minced fresh ginger
1 tbsp. sesame seeds

Combine all ingredients and mix well. Will keep in the fridge for two weeks. Stir before each use.

Endnotes

Preface

1   "Inspiration." Sept. 2012. Web. http://iheartinspiration.com/quotes/the-food-you-eat/

Chapter One: Tummy Tales . . .

2   "Hot Vegetarian Celebrities." *Squidoo*. Sept. 2012. Web. http://www.squidoo.com/vegetariancelebs

3   "Digestive Disorders." *John Hopkins Medicine Health Alerts*. Feb. 2013. Web. http://www.johnshopkinshealthalerts.com/alerts_index/digestive_health/19-1.html

4   "What is Irritable Bowel Syndrome? (IBS)." *Women's Health.Gov*. Feb. 2013. Web. http://www.womenshealth.gov/publications/our-publications/fact-sheet/irritable-bowel-syndrome.cfm

5   "Statistics." *Canadian Digestive Health Foundation*. 2013. Web. http://www.cdhf.ca/digestive-disorders/statistics.shtml

6   "U.S. and World Population Clocks." *United States Census Bureau*. Feb. 2013. Web. http://www.census.gov/main/www/popclock.html

Chapter Two: Digestion 101

7   "Small Intestine." *Wikipedia*. 2012. Web. http://en.wikipedia.org/wiki/Small_intestine

8   "Leaky Gut Syndrome." *Digestive Care Expert, Brenda Watson*. Feb. 2013. Web. http://www.brendawatson.com/digestive-conditions/leaky-gut/

9   "The Brain-Gut Connection." *Alternative Medicine Angel*. Feb. 2013. Web. http://altmedangel.com/gutbrain.htm

10   "Hypochlorhydria Screening Quiz: Low Stomach Acid Assessment." *About.Com: Alternative Health Medicine*. Feb. 2013. Web. http://altmedicine.about.com/library/weekly/bl_quiz_hypochlorhydria.htm

Chapter Three: The D.D. No One Wants Around

11   James E. Everhart, M.D., M.P.H. Chapter 1. "All Digestive Diseases." *The burden of digestive diseases in the United States*. US Department of Health and Human Services, Public Health Service, National Institutes of Health, National Institute of Diabetes and Digestive and Kidney Diseases. Washington, DC: US Government Printing Office, 2008; NIH Publication No. 09-6443. http://www3.niddk.nih.gov/Burden_of_Digestive_Diseases/index.shtml#CHAPTER1.

12   Campbell, T. Colin, PhD and Thomas M. Campbell, MD. *The China Study: Startling Implications for Diet, Weight-loss, and Long-Term Health*. Dallas, TX: Benbella Books, 2006, p. 76.

13   Ibid.

14   "Statistics." *Canadian Digestive Health Foundation*. 2012. Web. http://www.cdha.ca/digestive-disorders/statistics.shtml

15   "Irritable Bowel Syndrome." *The National Digestive Diseases Information Clearinghouse*. Feb. 2013. Web. http://digestive.niddk.nih.gov/ddiseases/pubs/ibs/

16   "Irritable Bowel Syndrome and Lactose Intolerance." *Livestrong.Com*. Feb. 2013. Web. http://www.livestrong.com/article/257849-irritable-bowel-syndrome-lactose-intolerance/

17   http://digestive.niddk.nih.gov/ddiseases/pubs/ibs/

18   "Irritable Bowel Syndrome." *Gastrointestinal Society: Canadian Society of Intestinal Research*. Feb. 2013. Web. http://www.badgut.org/information-centre/irritable-bowel-syndrome.html

19   "Irritable Bowel Syndrome." *Wikipedia*. Feb. 2013. Web. http://en.wikipedia.org/wiki/Irritable_bowel_syndrome

20   "Irritable Bowel Syndrome." *The National Digestive Diseases Information Clearinghouse*. Feb. 2013. Web. http://digestive.niddk.nih.gov/ddiseases/pubs/ibs/

21   Ibid

22   Homepage. *Canadian Digestive Health Foundation*. Feb. 2013. Web. www.cdhf.ca

23 "Statistics." *Canadian Digestive Health Foundation.* 2012. Web. http://www.cdha.ca/digestive-disorders/statistics.shtml

24 "Diverticulosis and Diverticulitis." *National Digestive Diseases Information Clearinghouse.* Feb. 2013. Web. http://digestive.niddk.nih.gov/ddiseases/pubs/diverticulosis/index.aspx

25 Ibid.

26 Ibid.

27 Hulse, Elliot. "Do You Know Your Sh*t? (Why I Look in the Toilet)" *Grow Stronger Blog.* Oct. 2012. Web. http://www.hulsestrength.com/sht-toilet/

28 "Diverticulitis." *Wikipedia.* 2012. Web. http://en.wikipedia.org/wiki/Diverticulitis

29 Ibid.

30 "Diverticulosis and Diverticulitis." *National Digestive Diseases Information Clearinghouse.* Feb. 2013. Web. http://digestive.niddk.nih.gov/ddiseases/pubs/diverticulosis/index.aspx

31 "Diverticulitis." Wikipedia. 2012. Web. http://en.wikipedia.org/wiki/Diverticulitis

32 Dr. Murphy, T. et al. "Diverticular Disease." *World Gastroenterology Organisation.* 2007. Web. http://www.worldgastroenterology.org/assets/downloads/en/pdf/guidelines/07_diverticular_disease.pdf

33 Ibid.

34 Homepage. *Canadian Digestive Health Foundation.* Feb. 2013. Web. www.cdhf.ca

35 "Diverticular Disease." *Canadian Digestive Health Foundation.* 2012. Web. http://www.cdhf.ca/digestive-disorders/statistics.shtml#diverticular

36 "Inflammatory Bowel Disease." *Wikipedia.* 2012. Web. http://en.wikipedia.org/wiki/Inflammatory_bowel_disease

37 "Crohn's Disease." *Canadian Digestive Health Foundation.* 2012. Web. http://www.cdhf.ca/digestive-disorders/crohns-disease.shtml

38 Homepage. *Crohn's and Colitis Foundation of America.* Feb. 2013. Web. http://www.ccfa.org/

39 "What is Crohn's Disease?" *Crohn's and Colitis Foundation of America.* Feb. 2013 Web. http://www.ccfa.org/what-are-crohns-and-colitis/what-is-crohns-disease/

40 "What is Ulcerative Colitis?" *Crohn's and Colitis Foundation of America.* Feb. 2013 Web. http://www.ccfa.org/what-are-crohns-and-colitis/what-is-ulcerative-colitis/

41   "Statistics." *Canadian Digestive Health Foundation.* 2012. Web. http://www.cdhf.ca/digestive-disorders/statistics.shtml

42   Roberts, Elizabeth. "Diets, diets, diets. . .What's an IBDer to do?" *HealthCentral.* Aug. 13, 2008. Web. http://www.healthcentral.com/ibd/c/2623/37082/diets-diets-diets-ibder/

43   Mitchell, Peter. "Carrot Juice and Crohn's Disease." *Livestrong.Com.* June. 2011. Web. http://www.livestrong.com/article/461333-carrot-juice-crohns-disease/

44   "Coeliac Disease." *Wikipedia.* 2012. Web. http://en.wikipedia.org/wiki/Celiac_disease

45   Lapid, Nancy. "How Common is Celiac Disease." *About.Com.* Nov. 2009. Web. http://celiacdisease.about.com/od/faqs/f/HowCommon.htm

46   "Coeliac Disease." Wikipedia. 2012. Web. http://en.wikipedia.org/wiki/Celiac_disease

47   "Celiac Disease Facts and Figures." *National Foundation for Celiac Awareness.* 2011. Web. http://www.celiaccentral.org/celiac-disease/facts-and-figures/

48   Ibid.

49   "Statistics." *Canadian Digestive Health Foundation.* 2012. Web. http://www.cdhf.ca/digestive-disorders/statistics.shtml

50   "GERD: Definition." *Mayo Clinic.* Feb. 2013. Web. http://www.mayoclinic.com/health/gerd/DS00967

51   "Signs and Symptoms of Acid Reflux." *Healthline.* June 30, 2012. Web. http://www.healthline.com/health/acid-reflux-symptoms

52   Homepage. *American Academy of Family Physicians.* Feb. 2013. Web. www.aafp.org

53   Scott, Mark, MD and Aimee R. Gelhot, Pharm.D. "Gastroesophageal Reflux Disease: Diagnosis and Management." *American Family Physician.* Mar. 1999. Web. http://www.aafp.org/afp/1999/0301/p1161.html

54   "Statistics." *Canadian Digestive Health Foundation.* 2012. Web. http://www.cdhf.ca/digestive-disorders/statistics.shtml

55   "Lactose Intolerance." *Canadian Digestive Health Foundation.* 2012. Web. http://www.cdhf.ca/digestive-disorders/lactose-intolerance.shtml

56   "Lactose Intolerance." *Ohio State Wexner Medical Center.* Feb. 2013. Web. http://medicalcenter.osu.edu/patientcare/healthcare_services/digestive_disorders/lactose_intolerance/Pages/index.aspx

57   "Statistics." *Canadian Digestive Health Foundation*. 2012. Web. http://www.cdhf.ca/digestive-disorders/statistics.shtml

Chapter Four: Inflammation Nation

58   Brazier, Brendan. *The Thrive Diet: The Whole Food Way to Losing Weight, Reducing Stress, and Staying Healthy for Life*. Philadelphia, PA: Da Capo Press, 2007, p. 47.

59   Carr, Kris. *Crazy, Sexy, Diet: Eat Your Veggies, Ignite Your Spark, and Live Like You Mean It!* Guildford, CT: Globe Pequot Press, 2011, p. 50.

60   "Is Cow's Milk Giving You Asthma?" *Food Matters*. Feb. 2013. Web. http://foodmatters.tv/articles-1/is-cows-milk-giving-you-asthma

61   "Food Allergy and Intolerance." *Better Health Channel*. Feb. 2013. Web. http://www.betterhealth.vic.gov.au/bhcv2/bhcarticles.nsf/pages/Food_allergy_and_intolerance

62   "Hippocrates." *GoodReads*. 2012. Web. http://www.goodreads.com/quotes/62262-let-food-be-thy-medicine-and-medicine-be-thy-food

Chapter Five: Healthcare 9-1-1

63   Foer, Jonathan Safran. *Eating Animals*. New York: Little, Brown, and Company, 2009, p. 141.

64   "Rates of Chronic Disease Expected to Rise Sharply." *American Association for Clinical Chemistry*. July 2009: Volume 35, Number 7. Web. http://www.aacc.org/publications/cln/2009/july/Pages/newsbrief0709.aspx#

65   Goldstein, Hesh. "Dairy: Beware of the Great White Hype (Opinion)" *Natural News.com* Oct. 2009. Web. http://www.naturalnews.com/027319_milk_dairy_Monsanto.html

66   Campbell, T. Colin, PhD and Thomas M. Campbell, MD. *The China Study: Startling Implications for Diet, Weight-loss, and Long-Term Health*. Dallas, TX: Benbella Books, 2006, p. 327.

67   Ibid. p. 329.

68   Ibid. p. 327.

69   Robbins, John. *No Happy Cows: Dispatches from the Frontlines of the Food Revolution*. San Francisco, CA: Conari Press, 2012, p. 141.

70   "Dean Ornish, MD." *Preventative Medicine Research Institute*. 2013. Web. http://www.pmri.org/dean_ornish.html

71   "Ornish Programs Reimbursed by Medicare." *Preventative Medicine Research Institute*. Feb. 2013. Web. http://www.pmri.org/certified_programs.html

72   "Protein Overload." *The McDougall Newsletter*. Jan. 2004, Vol. 3 No. 1. Web. http://www.drmcdougall.com/misc/2004nl/040100puproteinoverload.htm

73   Barnard, Dr. Neal. *Forks Over Knives: The Plant-Based Way to Health*. New York: The Experiment, LLC, 2011, p. 55.

Chapter Six: A Pitch for Vegetarianism

74   "Vegetarian Quotes." *Boston Vegetarian Society*. 2012. Web. http://www.bostonveg.org/quotes.html

75   Silverstone, Alicia. *The Kind Life*. 2012. Web. http://thekindlife.com

76   "Eat more Chicken, Fish, and Beans than Red Meat." *American Heart Association*. June 2012. Web. http://www.heart.org/HEARTORG/GettingHealthy/WeightManagement/LosingWeight/Eat-More-Chicken-Fish-and-Beans-than-Red-Meat_UCM_320278_Article.jsp

77   Mills, Milton R. MD. "The Comparative Anatomy of Eating." *VegSource.com*. 2012. Web. http://www.vegsource.com/news/2009/11/the-comparative-anatomy-of-eating.html

78   Knoff, Laura J. *The Whole-Food Guide to Overcoming Irritable Bowel Syndrome: Strategies and Recipes for Eating Well with IBS, Indigestion, and Other Digestive Disorders*. Oakland, CA: New Harbinger, 2010, p.34.

79   Campbell, T. Colin, PhD and Thomas M. Campbell, MD. *The China Study: Startling Implications for Diet, Weight-loss, and Long-Term Health*. Dallas, TX: Benbella Books, 2006, p. 88.

80   Epstein, Samuel S. M.D. "Monsanto's Genetically Modified Milk Ruled Unsafe by The United Nations." *PRNewswire*. Aug. 18. 1999. Web. http://www.preventcancer.com/publications/pdf/PR_Monsanto_aug1899.htm

81   Campbell, T. Colin, PhD and Thomas M. Campbell, MD. *The China Study: Startling Implications for Diet, Weight-loss, and Long-Term Health*. Dallas, TX: Benbella Books, 2006, p. 88.

82   Carlson-Rink, ND, RM, Cathy. "Preventing Osteoporosis." *Alive Magazine*. Web. http://www.alive.com/articles/view/19667/preventing_osteoporosis

83   "Environmental Chemicals and Breast Cancer Risk: Why is There Concern?" *Cornell University Program on Breast Cancer and*

Environmental Risk Factors in New York State (BCERF). May 2002. Web. http://envirocancer.cornell.edu/factsheet/general/fs45.chemical.pdf

84   Hyman, MD, Mark. "Dairy: 6 Reasons You Should Avoid It at All Costs or Why Following the USDA Food Pyramid Guidelines is Bad for Your Health (VIDEO)." *Huffpost Healthy Living*. http://www.huffingtonpost.com/dr-mark-hyman/dairy-free-dairy-6-reason_b_558876.html

85   O'Grady, Kathleen. "Early puberty for girls. The new 'normal' and why we need to be concerned." *Canadian Women's Health Network*. Fall/Winter 2008/09 Volume 11, Number 1. Web. http://www.cwhn.ca/en/node/39365

86   "Experts Probe Hospital Overcrowding," by Jeff Nagel, Abbotsford News, Feb. 9, 2012. Print.

87   Ibid.

88   Gardner, Amanda. "Bacteria Seen in Nearly Half of U.S. Meat." *CNN Health*. April 15, 2011. http://www.cnn.com/2011/HEALTH/04/15/bacteria.in.half.US.meat/index.html

89   News 1130. "Patients treated at Tim Hortons due to overcrowded ER." *News 1130*. March 2011. Web. http://www.news1130.com/news/local/article/190442--patients-treated-at-tim-hortons-due-to-overcrowded-er

90   "Quotations About Health." *The Quote Garden*. 2012. Web. http://www.quotegarden.com/health.html

91   Ibid.

92   "Bisphenol A." *Wikipedia*. 2012. Web. http://en.wikipedia.org/wiki/Bisphenol_A

93   Bisphenol-A (BPA)" *The New York Times*. July 17, 2012. Web. http://topics.nytimes.com/top/reference/timestopics/subjects/b/bisphenol_a/index.html

94   Lappé, Anna. "Small Planet Institute." *O Magazine*. June 2003. Print.

95   "Quotations About Health." *The Quote Garden*. 2012. Web. http://www.quotegarden.com/health.html

96   "2012 World Hunger and Poverty Facts and Statistics." *WorldHunger.org*. 2012. Web. http://www.worldhunger.org/articles/Learn/world%20hunger%20facts%202002.htm#Number_of_hungry_people_in_the_world

97   Homepage. *PETA*. 2012. Web. http://www.peta.org

98   Ladner, Peter. *The Urban Food Revolution: Changing the Way We Feed Cities*. Gabriola Island, BC: New Society Publishers, 2011, p.18.

99   Brazier, Brendan. *The Thrive Diet: The Whole Food Way to Losing Weight, Reducing Stress, and Staying Healthy for Life*. Philadelphia, PA: Da Capo Press, 2007, p. 93.

100   Mohr, Noam. "A New Global Warming Strategy: How Environmentalists are Overlooking Vegetarianism as the Most Effective Tool Against Climate Change in Our Lifetimes." *EarthSave*. Aug. 2005. Web. http://www.earthsave.org/globalwarming.htm

101   "Meat and the Environment." *PETA*. 2012. Web. http://www.peta.org/issues/animals-used-for-food/meat-and-environment.aspx

102   Foer, Jonathan Safran. *Eating Animals*. New York: Little, Brown, and Company, 2009, p. 103.

103   Homepage. *Sumas Mountain Farms*. Feb. 2013. Web. http://sumasmountainfarms.ca/

104   Homepage. *Farm Sanctuary*. Feb. 2013. Web. http://www.farmsanctuary.org/

105   Baur, Gene. *Farm Sanctuary: Changing Hearts and Minds about Animals and Food*. New York: Touchstone, 2008, p. 22.

106   Foer, Jonathan Safran. *Eating Animals*. New York: Little, Brown, and Company, 2009, p. 143.

107   "Chickens Used for Food." *PETA*. 2012. Web. http://www.peta.org/issues/animals-used-for-food/chickens.aspx

108   Hatfield, J.L. et al. "Swine Manure Management." Web. http://www.ars.usda.gov/is/np/agbyproducts/agbychap4.pdf

109   "Animal Waste Lagoon Factsheet." *SociallyResposibleAgriculture.org*. 2012. Web. http://www.sraproject.org/wp-content/uploads/2007/12/animalwastelagoonfactsheetnrdc.pdf

110   "Factsheet: Why Animal Waste Lagoons on Factory Farms should be Banned." (Adapted from "Cesspools of Shame", *National Resources Defense Council and Clean Water Network*. 2001.) Web. http://www.sraproject.org/wp-content/uploads/2007/12/whyanimalwastelagoonsonfactoryfarmsshouldbebanned.pdf

111   "Animal Waste Lagoon Factsheet." SociallyResposibleAgriculture.org. 2012. Web. http://www.sraproject.org/wp-content/uploads/2007/12/animalwastelagoonfactsheetnrdc.pdf

112   "For Your Health." *WhyVeg.com*. 2012. Web. http://whyveg.com/health/

113   MacKinnon, J.B. and Alisa Smith. *The 100-Mile Diet: A Year of Local Eating*. Random House of Canada, 2007, p.56.

114   Ladner, Peter. *The Urban Food Revolution: Changing the Way We Feed Cities.* Gabriola Island, BC: New Society Publishers, 2011, p. 10.

115   Stephens, Arran. *The Compassionate Diet: How What You Eat Can Change Your Life and Save the Planet.* New York: Rodale, 2011, p. 147.

116   Robbins, John. *The Food Revolution: How Your Diet Can Help Save Your Life and Our World.* San Francisco, CA: Conari Press, 2011, p. 290.

117   Campbell, T. Colin, PhD and Thomas M. Campbell, MD. *The China Study: Startling Implications for Diet, Weight-loss, and Long-Term Health.* Dallas, TX: Benbella Books, 2006, p. 305.

118   Foer, Jonathan Safran. *Eating Animals.* New York: Little, Brown, and Company, 2009, p. 1.

119   Ibid. p. 121.

120   Ibid. p. 131.

121   Stone, Gene, ed. *Forks Over Knives: The Plant-Based Way to Health.* New York: The Experiment, LLC, 2011, p. 4. Print.

122   Allen, Laura. "Senate Version of Egg Products Act Amendments Introduced." *Animal Law Coalition.* May 2012. Web. http://www.animallawcoalition.com/farm-animals/article/1679

123   "Factory Farming." *Farm Forward.* Feb. 2013. Web. http://www.farmforward.com/farming-forward/factory-farming

124   Stephens, Arran. *The Compassionate Diet: How What You Eat Can Change Your Life and Save the Planet.* New York: Rodale, 2011, p. 142.

125   "The Rotten Egg Industry." *Choose Veg.Com.* Feb. 2013. Web. http://www.chooseveg.com/eggs.asp

126   "Animal Disposition Reporting System." *The United States Department of Agriculture Food Safety and Inspection Service.* 2002. Web. http://www.fsis.usda.gov/science/Animal_Disposition_Reporting_System/index.asp

127   Lymbery, Philip. "Facts and Figures." *A Compassionate World.* May 2012. Web. http://www.acompassionateworld.org/facts-and-figures/

128   Foer, Jonathan Safran. *Eating Animals.* New York: Little, Brown, and Company, 2009, p. 48.

129   "Heritage." *Farm Forward.* Feb. 2013. Web. http://www.farmforward.com/features/heritage

130   "Food Myths." *State of Alaska Food Safety and Sanitation Program.* Feb. 2013. Web. http://www.dec.alaska.gov/eh/fss/consumers/food_myths.htm

131   Foer, Jonathan Safran. Eating Animals. New York: Little, Brown, and Company, 2009, p. 58.

132   Ibid. p. 19.

133   Ibid. p. 43.

134   Stephens, Arran. *The Compassionate Diet: How What You Eat Can Change Your Life and Save the Planet.* New York: Rodale, 2011, p. 149.

135   United States. *United States Environmental Protection Agency.* "What's the Problem?" Web. http://www.epa.gov/region9/animalwaste/problem. html

136   Wood, Richard R. and Sosa, Meryl Camin. "The Comments of Food Animal Concerns Trust in response to the Draft Preliminary Food Safety Strategic Plan for Public Review." *FACT.* Feb. 2000. Web. http://www. fda.gov/ohrms/dockets/dockets/97n0074/c000224.pdf

137   "Did you know . . .? Fact and Figures about Water Footprints and Virtual Water." *UNESCO.* July 2011. Web. http://www.unesco.org/water/ news/newsletter/252.shtml#know

138   "Go Vegetarian." *Greenpeace.* July 2007. Web. http://www.greenpeace. org/usa/en/multimedia/goodies/green-guide/green-lifestyle/go-vegetarian/

139   Food and Agriculture Organization of the United Nation. "Livestock's Role in Climate Change and Air Pollution." *Livestock's Long Shadow-Environmental Issues and Opinions.* Rome: 2006. Web. ftp://ftp.fao.org/ docrep/fao/010/a0701e/a0701e00.pdf

140   Ibid.

Chapter Seven: Filthy Food

141   "Jack in the Box." *Wikipedia.* 2012. Web. http://en.wikipedia.org/wiki/ Jack_in_the_Box

142   SafeFood Rapid Response Network. "The Hudson Foods Recall . . . the Rest of the Story." *SafeFood News.* 1997. Web. http://www.ext. colostate.edu/safefood/newsltr/v2n1s02.html

143   Mokhiber, Russell and Robert Weissman. "Ball Park Franks Fiasco: 21 Dead, $200,000 Fine." *Common Dreams: Building Progressive Company.* July 2001. Web. http://www.commondreams.org/ views01/0726-04.htm

144   "2008 Canada Listeriosis Outbreak." *Wikipedia.* 2012. Web. http:// en.wikipedia.org/wiki/2008_Canada_listeriosis_outbreak

145   "XL Foods Faces New Lawsuits from B.C .Residents." *CBC News*. Oct. 17, 2012. Web. http://www.cbc.ca/news/canada/story/2012/10/17/xl-foods-beef-recall-expands.html

146   "Food Myths." *State of Alaska Food Safety and Sanitation Program*. Feb. 2013. Web. http://www.dec.alaska.gov/eh/fss/consumers/food_myths.htm

147   Segarra, Alejandro E. and Jean M. Rawson. "Mad Cow Disease: Agricultural Issues." *U.S. Department of State*. March 2001. Web. http://fpc.state.gov/6121.htm

148   "U.S. Beef Industry Facts." *Center for Food Safety*. 2013. Web. http://www.centerforfoodsafety.org/campaign/food-safety/mad-cow-disease/other-resources/a-consumers-guide-to-mad-cow-disease/u-s-beef-industry-facts/

149   Kanade, Shrinivas. "Mad Cow Disease Facts." *Buzzle*. 2013. Web. http://www.buzzle.com/articles/mad-cow-disease-facts.html

150   Robbins, John. *The Food Revolution: How Your Diet Can Help Save Your Life and Our World*. San Francisco, CA: Conari Press, 2011, p. 116.

151   "Fact Sheet: Irradiation and Food Safety." *United States Department of Agriculture Food Safety and Inspection Service*. 2013. Web. http://www.fsis.usda.gov/Fact_Sheets/Irradiation_and_Food_Safety/index.asp#3

152   "Food Irradiation." *Canadian Food Inspection Agency*. 2012. Web. http://www.inspection.gc.ca/food/consumer-centre/food-safety-tips/labelling-food-packaging-and-storage/irradiation/eng/1332358607968/1332358680017

153   "Fact Sheet: Irradiation and Food Safety." *United States Department of Agriculture Food Safety and Inspection Service*. 2013. Web. http://www.fsis.usda.gov/Fact_Sheets/Irradiation_and_Food_Safety/index.asp#3

154   "Food Irradiation." *Canadian Food Inspection Agency*. 2012. Web. http://www.inspection.gc.ca/food/consumer-centre/food-safety-tips/labelling-food-packaging-and-storage/irradiation/eng/1332358607968/1332358680017

155   Stephens, Arran. *The Compassionate Diet: How What You Eat Can Change Your Life and Save the Planet*. New York: Rodale, 2011, p. 103.

156   "Monsanto." *Wikipedia*. 2012. Web. http://en.wikipedia.org/wiki/Monsanto

157   Embree, Bryan. "For presentation to the House of Commons Standing Committee on Health Hearing on the Labelling of GM Foods." *Ontario Public Health Association Workgroups*. 2002. Web. http://www.opha.on.ca/resources/docs/foodbiotech/houseofcommons.html

158   Smith, Jeffrey M. *Genetic Roulette: The Documented Health Risks of Genetically Engineered Foods.* Written and Directed by Smith, Jeffrey M. 2012. DVD.

159   Embree, Bryan. "For presentation to the House of Commons Standing Committee on Health Hearing on the Labelling of GM Foods." *Ontario Public Health Association Workgroups.* 2002. Web. http://www.opha. on.ca/resources/docs/foodbiotech/houseofcommons.html

160   "Monsanto." *Wikipedia.* 2012. Web. http://en.wikipedia.org/wiki/ Monsanto

161   *Genetic Roulette: The Documented Health Risks of Genetically Engineered Foods.* Written and Directed by Smith, Jeffrey M. 2012. DVD.

162   "Genetically Modified Maize." *Wikipedia.* 2012. Web. http:// en.wikipedia.org/wiki/Genetically_modified_maize

163   Mercola, Dr. "How Can the Wealthiest Industrialized Nation by the Sickest?" *Mercola.com.* 2012. Web. http://articles.mercola.com/sites/ articles/archive/2012/09/15/genetic-roulette-gmo-documentary.aspx

164   "Leaky Gut Syndrome." *Wikipedia.* 2012. Web. http://en.wikipedia.org/ wiki/Leaky_gut_syndrome

165   "Genetically Engineered Crops." *Center for Food Safety.* 2013. Web. http://www.centerforfoodsafety.org/campaign/genetically-engineered-food/crops/

166   Robbins, John. *No Happy Cows: Dispatches from the Frontlines of the Food Revolution.* San Francisco, CA: Conari Press, 2012, p. 53.

167   "Advertisement: DDT is Good For Me." *International Society for Environmental Ethics.* June 2011. Web. http://enviroethics. org/2011/06/18/animation-ddd-is-good-for-me/

168   "Probiotics Found to Help Your Gut's Immune System." *Mercola. Com.* July 2008. Web. http://articles.mercola.com/sites/articles/ archive/2008/07/05/probiotics-found-to-help-your-gut-s-immune-system. aspx

169   Foer, Jonathan Safran. *Eating Animals.* New York: Little, Brown, and Company, 2009, p. 140.

Chapter Eight: Chemically Speaking

170   "Food." Merriam-Webster Dictionary. 2012. Web. http://www.merriam-webster.com/dictionary/food

171   "Nutraceutical." *Wikipedia*. 2012. Web. http://en.wikipedia.org/wiki/Nutraceutical

172   Pollan, Michael. *In Defense of Food: An Eater's Manifesto*. New York: Penguin, 2008, p. 27.

173   Brazier, Brendan. *The Thrive Diet: The Whole Food Way to Losing Weight, Reducing Stress, and Staying Healthy for Life*. Philadelphia, PA: Da Capo Press, 2007, p. 37.

174   John Robbins, *The Food Revolution: How Your Diet Can Help Save Your Life and Our World*. San Francisco, CA: Conari Press, 2011, p. 12.

175   "Generally Recognized as Safe." *United States Food and Drug Administration*. 2012. Web. http://www.fda.gov/Food/FoodIngredientsPackaging/GenerallyRecognizedasSafeGRAS/default.htm

176   "Coke, Pepsi to Change Caramel Coloring Recipes." *Fox News*. March 2012. Web. http://www.foxnews.com/health/2012/03/09/coke-pepsi-to-change-caramel-coloring-recipes/

177   Sherpa, Coupon. "Top 15 Chemical Additives in Your Food." *Phys.org*. Jan. 2010. Web. http://phys.org/news183110037.html

178   Ibid.

179   Ibid.

180   Ibid.

181   Ibid.

182   Ibid.

183   Ibid.

184   Ibid.

185   Ibid.

186   Ibid.

187   Ibid.

188   Ibid.

189   Ibid.

190   Ibid.

191   Carr, Kris. *Crazy, Sexy, Diet: Eat Your Veggies, Ignite Your Spark, and Live Like You Mean It!* Guilford, CT: Globe Pequot Press, 2011, p.79.

192   Homepage. *David Suzuki Foundation*. 2013. Web. www.davidsuzuki.org

193   "Health." *David Suzuki Foundation*. 2012. Web. http://www.davidsuzuki.org/issues/health/science/toxics/dirty-dozen-cosmetic-chemicals

194   "About Us." *David Suzuki Foundation.* 2012. Web. http://www.
davidsuzuki.org/issues/health/science/toxics/dirty-dozen-cosmetic-
chemicals

195   "Dirty Dozen Cosmetic Chemicals to Avoid." *David Suzuki
Foundation.* 2012. Web. http://www.davidsuzuki.org/issues/health/
science/toxics/dirty-dozen-cosmetic-chemicals/

196   Ibid.

197   Jonathan Bailor. "57 Sugars that are Destroying Your Health."
DietsinReview.com. 2012. Web. http://us.m.yahoo.com/w/legobpengine/
lifestyles/blogs/healthy-living/57-sugars-destroying-health-151700936.
html?.b=index&.ts=1351637258&.intl=US&.lang=en&.
ysid=XOL6vPDt_5Sksoid0ZqVEDOA

198   McKenzie, Brian and Melanie Rapino. "Commuting in the United
States: 2009." *United States Census Bureau.* Sept. 2011. Web. http://
www.census.gov/prod/2011pubs/acs-15.pdf

199   Herr, Norman, Ph.D. "Television and Health." *California State
University: Sourcebook.* 2007. Web. http://www.csun.edu/science/health/
docs/tv&health.html

200   "Diabetes Public Health Resource." *Centers for Disease Control and
Prevention.* 2013. Web. http://www.cdc.gov/diabetes/projects/cda2.htm

201   Pollan, Michael. *In Defense of Food: An Eater's Manifesto.* New York:
Penguin, 2008, p. 148.

Chapter Nine: Get Wet!

202   Q, Shi et al. "Regulation of Vascular Endothelial Growth Factor
Expression by Acidosis in Human Cancer Cells." *Department of
Gastrointestinal Medical Oncology, The University of Texas.* Anderson
Cancer Center. *PubMed Central.* June 2001. Web. http://europepmc.org/
abstract/MED/11439338/reload=0;jsessionid=VDRg8CRJbklVBaKwH6
sE.4

203   "Alkaline Water: The Battle Over pH." *Organic Lives.* Jan. 2012. Web.
http://organiclives.ca/_blog/OrganicLives_Blog/post/Alkaline_Water_
The_Battle_Over_pH/

204   "Testing of Various Brands of Bottled Water and Municipal Tap Water."
Alkaline Water Plus. 2013. Web. http://www.alkalinewaterplus.com/
Popular-Water-Brands-PH-and-ORP

205   Perez, Ava. "How to Alkalize Foods and pH Levels." *eHow.* 2012. Web.
http://www.ehow.com/how_7197537_alkalize-foods-ph-levels.html

206   "The Acid/Alkaline Foods List." *Angelfire*. 2012. Web. http://www. angelfire.com/az/sthurston/acid_alkaline_foods_list.html

207   "The Water in You." *The USGS Water Science School*. 2013. Web. http://ga.water.usgs.gov/edu/propertyyou.html

208   "Water—a Vital Nutrient." *Better Health Channel*. 2013. Web. http://www.betterhealth.vic.gov.au/bhcv2/bhcarticles.nsf/pages/Water_a_vital_nutrient

209   Ibid.

Chapter Ten: Serious Solutions for Happy Digestion

210   Mitchell, Joni. "Big Yellow Taxi." *Joni Mitchell*. 2012. Web. http://jonimitchell.com/music/song.cfm?id=208

211   "Why Organic?" *Green Earth Organics*. 2012. Web. http://seatosky. greenearthorganics.com/whyorganic/

212   Tawse, Sylvia. "Ten Reasons Why You Should Eat Organic Food." *Green Earth Organics*. (Excerpted from Organic Times, Spring 1992) 2013. Web. https://seatosky.greenearthorganics.com/whyorganic/

213   "When Should You Buy Organic?" *Environmental Working Group*. 2012. Web. http://www.ewg.org/release/when-should-you-buy-organic

214   Ibid.

215   "Health Benefits of Phytonutrients." *Your Self Centre*. Jan. 2011. Web. http://yourselfcentre.wordpress.com/2011/01/04/health-benefits-of-phytonutrients/

216   Dolson, Laura. "Eat Your Colors! (All About Phytonutrients)" *Cruzio*. Dec. 2004. Web. http://members.cruzio.com/~dolson/healthtips/colors.html

217   Ibid.

218   "Vitamin C Benefits." 2012. Web. http://www.vitamincbenefits.org/

219   "Lutein." *Muscle and Strength*. 2012. Web. http://www.muscleandstrength.com/supplements/ingredients/lutein.html

220   Dolson, Laura. "Eat Your Colors! (All About Phytonutrients)" *Cruzio*. Dec. 2004. Web. http://members.cruzio.com/~dolson/healthtips/colors.html

221   "Position of the American Dietetic Association and Dieticians of Canada: Vegetarian Diets." *Journal of the American Dietetic Association.* June 2003, Volume 103, Number 6. Print.

222   "Beginning Food Combining." *Health Source.* 2013. Web. http://www.trustedhands.com/fcintro.html

223   MacKinnon, J.B. and Alisa Smith. *The 100-Mile Diet: A Year of Local Eating.* Toronto, ON: Random House, 2007, p.3.

224   Miller, David Niven. "Sprouting." *Grow Youthful.* 2013. Web. http://www.growyouthful.com/recipes/sprouts.php

225   Brazier, Brendan. *The Thrive Diet: The Whole Food Way to Losing Weight, Reducing Stress, and Staying Healthy for Life.* Philadelphia, PA: Da Capo Press, 2007, p. 23.

226   Knoff, Laura. *The Whole-Food Guide to Overcoming Irritable Bowel Syndrome: Strategies and Recipes for Eating Well With IBS, Indigestion, and Other Digestive Disorders.* New Harbinger Publications, 2010, p 48.

227   Halpern, Marc. "Panchakarma: The Ayurvedic Science of Detoxification and Rejuvenation." *California College of Ayurveda.* 2012. Web. http://www.ayurvedacollege.com/articles/drhalpern/Panchakarma_Detoxification_Rejuvenation

228   Ibid.

Chapter Eleven: Food Rules

229   Pollan, Michael. *In Defense of Food: An Eater's Manifesto.* New York: Penguin, 2008, p.1.

230   "Vegetarian Diets." American Heart Association. 2013. Web. http://www.heart.org/HEARTORG/GettingHealthy/NutritionCenter/Vegetarian-Diets_UCM_306032_Article.jsp

231   "Protein." *Wikipedia.* 2013. Web. http://en.wikipedia.org/wiki/Protein_(nutrient)

232   "Amino Acid." *Wikipedia.* 2012. Web. http://en.wikipedia.org/wiki/Amino_acid

233   Hever, Julieanna. "3 Myths about Protein and a Plant-Based Diet." *VegNews.* July 2012. Web. http://vegnews.com/articles/page.do?catId=7&pageId=4753

234   "12 Frequently Asked Questions about the Vegetarian Diet." *Ask Dr. Sears.* 2013. Web. http://www.askdrsears.com/topics/family-nutrition/vegetarian-diets/12-frequently-asked-questions-about-vegetarian-diet

235   "Veganism and the Issue of Protein." *People for the Ethical Treatment of Animals*. 2013. Web. http://www.peta.org/issues/animals-used-for-food/veganism-and-the-issue-of-protein.aspx

236   Pollan, Michael. *In Defense of Food: An Eater's Manifesto*. New York: Penguin, 2008, p.109.

237   "Omega-3 Fatty Acid." *Wikipedia*. 2012. Web. http://en.wikipedia.org/wiki/Omega-3_fatty_acid

238   Iliades, MD, Chris. "Essential Vitamins for Digestive Health." *Everyday Health*. 2012. Web. http://www.everydayhealth.com/digestive-health/essential-vitamins-for-digestive-health.aspx

239   Knoff, Laura. *The Whole-Food Guide to Overcoming Irritable Bowel Syndrome: Strategies and Recipes for Eating Well With IBS, Indigestion, and Other Digestive Disorders*. New Harbinger Publications, 2010, pg. 42

240   Mangels, PhD, RD, Reid. (From Simply Vegan 5th Edition.) "Iron in the Vegan Diet." *The Vegetarian Resource Group*. 2013. Web. http://www.vrg.org/nutrition/iron.php

241   "Iron." *University of Maryland Medical Center*. 2011. Web. http://www.umm.edu/altmed/articles/iron-000309.htm

242   "Chemicals in Meat Cooked at High Temperatures and Cancer Risk." *National Cancer Institute*. 2010. Web. http://www.cancer.gov/cancertopics/factsheet/Risk/cooked-meats

243   Campbell, Ph.D, T. Colin. Animal vs. Plant Protein. *T. Colin Campbell Foundation*. 2008. Web. http://www.tcolincampbell.org/courses-resources/article/animal-vs-plant-protein/

244   "Vitamin Supplement Fact Sheet: Vitamin B12." *Office of Dietary Supplements: National Institutes of Health*. 2013. Web. http://ods.od.nih.gov/factsheets/VitaminB12-HealthProfessional/

245   Campbell, T. Colin, PhD and Thomas M. Campbell, MD. *The China Study: Startling Implications for Diet, Weight-loss, and Long-Term Health*. Dallas, TX: Benbella Books, 2006, p. 92.

246   Homepage. *Earthsave*. 2012. Web. http://www.earthsave.org/about1.html

247   Silverstone, Alicia. *The Kind Diet: A Simple Guide to Feeling Great, Losing Weight, and Saving the Planet*. New York: Rodale, 2009. p. 131.

Chapter Twelve: Get Healthy, Feel Beautiful

248   "Bob Marley Quotes." *Goodreads*. 2012. Web. http://www.goodreads.com/quotes/93997-love-the-life-you-live-live-the-life-you-love

249   Esselstyn, Dr. Caldwell JR, MD. *The China Study: Startling Implications for Diet, Weight-loss, and Long-Term Health*. Dallas, TX: Benbella Books, 2006, p. 326.

250   "Tax 'Toxic' Sugar, Doctors Urge: Age Restriction on Sugary Drinks Proposed." *CBC News*. Feb. 2012. Web. http://www.cbc.ca/news/health/story/2012/02/01/sugar-toxic-regulate.html

251   Baur, Gene. *Farm Sanctuary: Changing Hearts and Minds about Animals and Food*. New York: Touchstone, 2008, p. 222.

252   Robbins, John. *No Happy Cows: Dispatches from the Frontlines of the Food Revolution*. San Francisco, CA: Conari Press, 2012, p. 66.

About the Author

Jennifer Browne completed her Bachelor of Arts Degree in English Literature at the University of the Fraser Valley and has a Certificate in Plant-Based Nutrition from eCornell University. Although diagnosed with IBS in 2001, she has been symptom-free since the fall of 2010, which coincides with her adoption of a plant-based diet. Jennifer is an advocate for nutrition education, a member of EarthSave, and a member of CETFA (Canadians for the Ethical Treatment of Food Animals). She lives with her husband and three children just outside of Vancouver, British Columbia, and can be found munching on garlic-stuffed olives at www.jenniferbrowne. org.

She is currently working on *Happy Healthy Gut Foods: A Plant-Based Collection that Your Gut Will Love.*

Further Reading and Other Resources

Although I used most of these resources to help me write this book, I still refer to many of them on an ongoing basis. The list of further reading and documentary videos will only help you better formulate your own personal opinion regarding food, and what it means for your health, and the health of your family. I hope you don't stop investigating here; keep on with your food education so that you feel strong and confident with every bite of every food you choose to put into your mouth.

Books

- Barnard, Neal, M.D. *Foods that Fight Pain: Revolutionary New Strategies for Maximum Pain Relief.* New York: Random House, 1998.
- Barnouin, Kim and Rory Freeman. *Skinny Bitch: A No-Nonsense, Tough-Love Guide for Saavy Girls Who Want to Stop Eating Crap and Start Looking Fabulous.* Running Press, 2005.
- Baur, Gene. *Farm Sanctuary: Changing Hearts and Minds about Animals and Food.* New York: Touchstone, 2008.

- Brazier, Brendan. *The Thrive Diet: The Whole Food Way to Losing Weight, Reducing Stress, and Staying Healthy for Life.* Philadelphia, PA: Da Capo Press, 2007.
- Campbell, T. Colin, PhD and Thomas M. Campbell, MD. *The China Study: Startling Implications for Diet, Weight-loss, and Long-Term Health.* Dallas, TX: Benbella Books, 2006.
- Carr, Kris. *Crazy, Sexy, Diet: Eat Your Veggies, Ignite Your Spark, and Live Like You Mean It!* Guildford, CT: Globe Pequot Press, 2011.
- Foer, Jonathan Safran. *Eating Animals.* New York: Little, Brown, and Company, 2009.
- Freston, Kathy. *Veganist: Lose Weight, Get Healthy, Change the World.* New York: Weinstein Books, 2011.
- Knoff, Laura. *The Whole-Food Guide to Overcoming Irritable Bowel Syndrome: Strategies and Recipes for Eating Well With IBS, Indigestion, and Other Digestive Disorders.* New Harbinger Publications, 2010.
- Kotsopoulos, Peggy. *Must Have Been Something I Ate: The Simple Connection Between What You Eat and How You Look and Feel.* Coquitlam, BC: Oceanside Publishing INK, 2011.
- Ladner, Peter. *The Urban Food Revolution: Changing the Way We Feed Cities.* Gabriola Island, BC: New Society Publishers, 2011.
- MacKinnon, J.B. and Alisa Smith. *The 100-Mile Diet: A Year of Local Eating.* Canada: Random House, 2007.
- McDougall, Dr. John A. *Dr. McDougall's Digestive Tune-Up.* Summertown, TN: Book Publishing Company, 2006.
- McKeith, Dr. Jillian. *You Are What You Eat: The Plan That Will Change Your Life.* New York: Penguin, 2005.

- Pollan, Michael. *In Defense of Food: An Eater's Manifesto*. New York: Penguin, 2008.
- Pollan, Michael. *The Omnivore's Dilemma: A Natural History of Four Meals*. New York: Penguin, 2007.
- Porter, Jessica. *The Hip-Chick's Guide to Macrobiotics: A Philosophy for Achieving a Radiant Mind and Fabulous Body*. New York: Penguin, 2004.
- Robbins, John. *Diet for a New America: How Your Food Choices Affect Your Health, Happiness and the Future Of Life on Earth*. 1987.
- Robbins, John. *The Food Revolution: How Your Diet Can Help Save Your Life and Our World*. San Francisco, CA: Conari Press, 2011.
- Robbins, John. *No Happy Cows: Dispatches from the Frontlines of the Food Revolution*. San Francisco, CA: Conari Press, 2012.
- Silverstone, Alicia. *The Kind Diet: A Simple Guide to Feeling Great, Losing Weight, and Saving the Planet*. New York: Rodale, 2009.
- Smith, Jeffrey M. *Genetic Roulette: The Documented Health Risks of Genetically Engineered Foods*. Chelsea Green Publishing, 2007.
- Stephens, Arran. *The Compassionate Diet: How What You Eat Can Change Your Life and Save the Planet*. New York: Rodale, 2011.
- Stone, Gene, ed. *Forks Over Knives: The Plant-Based Way to Health*. New York: The Experiment, LLC, 2011.

Recipe Books

- Parragon Publishing. *Vegetarian*. Bath, UK: Parragon Publishing, 2009.

- Swanson, Heidi. *Super Natural Cooking: Five Ways to Incorporate Whole and Natural Ingredients into Your Cooking*. New York: Random House, 2007.
- Tal, Ruth. *Refresh*. Mississauga, ON: John Wiley & Sons, Canada, 2007.

Videos

- *Death on a Factory Farm* (2009). Directed by Tom Simon and Sarah Teale.
- *Forks Over Knives* (2011). Written and directed by Lee Fulkerson.
- *Food, Inc.* (2009). Directed by Robert Kenner. Written by Robert Kenner, Kim Roberts, and Elise Pearlstein.
- *Genetic Roulette: The Documented Health Risks of Genetically Engineered Foods*: A film by Jeffrey M. Smith. Narrated by Lisa Oz.
- *Super Size Me* (2004). Written and directed by Morgan Spurlock.
- *The World According to Monsanto* (2008). Directed by Marie-Monique Robin.
- *Vegucated* (2010). Written and directed by Marisa Miller Wolfson.

Websites

- Cage Free: www.choosecagefree.ca. Find out where to purchase eggs from hens that are free from battery cages.
- Canadian Digestive Health Foundation: http://www.cdhf.ca/main.php.
- National Digestive Diseases Information Clearinghouse: http://digestive.niddk.nih.gov/index.aspx.
- Canadians for the Ethical Treatment of Food Animals: www.cetfa.com.

- Canadian Society of Intestinal Research: www.ibsgroup. org.
- EarthSave: www.earthsave.ca (Canada) or http:// earthsave.org (United States)
- Eat Wild! www.eatwild.com. A website that locates 100% certified organic, SPCA -approved, and/or grass-fed and finished farms in your area. (Canada and U.S.)
- GMO Shopping Guide: www.nongmoshoppingguide. com. A website that will make your life easier when trying to avoid GMOs.
- Jennifer Browne: www.jenniferbrowne.org
- People for the Ethical Treatment of Animals: www.peta. org.
- Whole Foods Market: www.wholefoods.com. Various locations available throughout Canada and the U.S.

Index

X

Y